MPR

Medical Pocket Reference

ANTI-INFECTIVE DRUGS

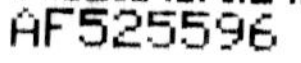

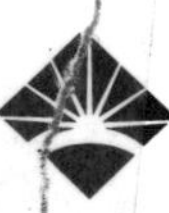

LIPPINCOTT WILLIAMS & WILKINS
A **Wolters Kluwer** Company
Philadelphia • Baltimore • New York • London
Buenos Aires • Hong Kong • Sydney • Tokyo

Staff

Publisher
Judy Schilling McCann, RN, MSN

Editorial Director
William J. Kelly

Senior Art Director
Arlene Putterman

Art Director
Elaine Kasmer

Clinical Manager
Eileen Cassin Gallen, RN, BSN

Drug Information Editor
Melissa M. Devlin, PharmD

Associate Editor
Christiane L. Brownell

Editors
Catherine E. Harold, Carol Turkington

Clinical Project Editor
Minh N. Luu, RN, BSN, JD

Clinical Editors
Lisa M. Bonsall, RN, MSN, CRNP;
Christine M. Damico, RN, MSN, CPNP

Copy Editors
Caryl Knutsen, Beth Pitcher

Electronic Production Services
Diane Paluba (manager),
Donald G. Knauss (project manager)
Joyce Rossi Biletz (senior desktop assistant)

Manufacturing
Patricia K. Dorshaw (manager),
Beth Janae Orr (book production manager)

Editorial Assistants
Danielle J. Barsky, Carol A. Caputo,
Arlene P. Claffee

Indexer
Deborah K. Tourtlotte

For information, write Lippincott Williams & Wilkins, 1111 Bethlehem Pike, P.O. Box 908, Springhouse, PA 19477-0908.

Visit our Web site at eDrugInfo.com

ISBN 1-58255-221-5
MPRAD—D N
05 04 03 02 10 9 8 7 6 5 4 3 2 1

Library of Congress Cataloging-in-Publication Data

Medical pocket reference : anti-infective drugs.
p.;cm.
Includes index.
1. Anti-infective agents—Handbooks, manuals, etc. 2. Communicable diseases—Treatment—Handbooks, manuals, etc. 3. Nursing—Handbooks, manuals, etc.
[DNLM: 1. Anti-Infective Agents—Handbooks. 2. Infection—drug therapy—Handbooks. QV 39 M4892 2003] I. Title: Anti-infective drugs. II. Lippincott Williams & Wilkins.
RM267 .M425 2003
616.9'0461—dc21 2002013633
ISBN 1-58255-221-5 (pbk.:alk. paper)

Contents

How to use this book

Medical Pocket Reference: Anti-Infective Drugs is designed to help you find essential drug information quickly. A list of all the abbreviations used in the drug entries appears first. Then come the entries organized alphabetically by generic name. Next to each generic name, you'll find common trade names.

The first column in each drug entry shows the drug's pharmacologic class and (after the semicolon) the therapeutic class. These are followed by the pregnancy risk category and, where applicable, controlled substance schedule.

Pregnancy risk categories parallel those assigned by the Food and Drug Administration to reflect a drug's potential to cause birth defects.

- A: Adequate studies in pregnant women have failed to show a risk to the fetus.
- B: Animal studies haven't shown a risk to the fetus, but controlled studies haven't been conducted in pregnant women; or animal studies have shown an adverse effect on the fetus, but adequate studies in pregnant women haven't shown a fetal risk.
- C: Animal studies have shown an adverse effect on the fetus, but adequate studies haven't been conducted in humans. The benefits may be acceptable despite potential risks.
- D: The drug may pose risks to the human fetus, but potential benefits may be acceptable despite the risks.
- X: Studies in animals or humans show fetal abnormalities, or reports of adverse reactions indicate evidence of fetal risk. The risks involved clearly outweigh the potential benefits.
- NR: Not rated.

Drugs regulated under the Controlled Substances Act of 1970 are divided into the following schedules:

- I: High abuse potential, no accepted medical use
- II: High abuse potential, severe dependence liability
- III: Less abuse potential than schedule II drugs, moderate dependence liability
- IV: Less abuse potential than schedule III drugs, limited dependence liability
- V: Limited abuse potential.

The second column lists how the drug is available—its preparations and dosage strengths.

The third column covers major indications and the most common dosages ordered for a particular drug. In this column, the multiplication symbol (×) is used for the word *for* to save space. Dosage adjustments are listed at the end of this section, when applicable.Symbols in the text indicate Canadian drugs (◆) and off-label uses (◇).

Appendices include therapeutic monitoring guidelines, a table comparing penicillins, a table comparing cephalosporins, and a list of dialyzable anti-infectives.

The index lists trade names, indications, pharmacologic classes, and therapeutic classes.

Guide to abbreviations

ABG	arterial blood gases
ac	before meals
ACE	angiotensin-converting enzyme
ADHD	attention-deficit hyperactivity disorder
admin	administration
AIDS	acquired immunodeficiency syndrome
ALL	acute lymphocytic leukemia
ALT	alanine aminotransferase
am	morning
amp	ampule
amt	amount
aPTT	activated partial thromboplastin time
ASAP	as soon as possible
AST	aspartate aminotransferase
ATC	around-the-clock
bid	twice a day
BM	bowel movement
BMT	bone marrow transplantation
BP	blood pressure
BPH	benign prostatic hyperplasia
buff	buffered
BUN	blood urea nitrogen
CA	cancer
CAD	coronary artery disease
capl	caplet
caps	capsule
CBC	complete blood count
CHD	coronary heart disease
chemo	chemotherapy
chew	chewable
CMV	cytomegalovirus
conc	concentrated
cont	continue, continuous
contr-rel	controlled-release
COPD	chronic obstructive pulmonary disease
CrCl	creatinine clearance
CSF	cerebrospinal fluid
CSS	Controlled Substance Schedule
CV	cardiovascular
CVA	cerebrovascular accident
d	day
decr	decrease
del-rel	delayed-release
dil	diluted, dilution
div	divided
dl	deciliter
DM	diabetes mellitus
DVT	deep vein thrombosis
ECG	echocardiogram
EEG	electroencephalogram
efferv	effervescent
elix	elixir
ent	enteric
equiv	equivalent
ET	endotracheal
eval	evaluation
exacer	exacerbation
exam	examination
ext-rel	extended-release
fib	fibrillation
g	gram
GERD	gastroesophageal reflux disease
GGT	gamma-glutamyl transpeptidase
GI	gastrointestinal

gram-neg	gram-negative
gram-pos	gram-positive
gtt	drop
GU	genitourinary
gyn	gynecologic
h	hour
H_2O	water
Hct	hematocrit
HF	heart failure
Hgb	hemoglobin
HBV	Hepatitis B virus
HIV	human immunodeficiency virus
HMG-CoA	3-hydroxy-methylglutaryl coenzyme A
hs	at bedtime
HSV	herpes simplex virus
Htn	hypertension
IBS	irritable bowel syndrome
IM	intramuscular
immed	immediate
incr	increase
inf	infusion
infect	infection
inhal	inhalant, inhalation
inhib	inhibitor
inj	injection
INR	international normalized ratio
intraop	intraoperative
intrav	intravaginally
IOP	intraocular pressure
IPPB	intermittent positive-pressure breathing
IU	international unit
IV	intravenous
kg	kilogram
L	liter
LDH	lactate dehydrogenase
liq	liquid
m^2	square meter
MAC	*Mycobacterium avium* complex
maint	maintenance
MAO	monoamine oxidase
max	maximum
mcg	microgram
med	medication
mEq	milliequivalent
mg	milligram
mgt	management
MI	myocardial infarction
min	minute
ml	milliliter
mo	month
mol	molecular
MRSA	methicillin-resistant staphylococcus aureus
MS	multiple sclerosis
MSSA	methicillin-susceptible staphylococcus aureus
NaCl	sodium chloride
neb	nebulizer
NG	nasogastric
NSS	normal saline solution
NSAID	nonsteroidal anti-inflammatory drug
OA	osteoarthritis
OC	oral contraceptive
oint	ointment
OM	otitis media
ophth	ophthalmic
oz	ounce
PAC	premature atrial contraction
PAT	paroxysmal atrial tachycardia

pc	after meals
PCN	penicillin
PE	pulmonary embolism
ped	pediatric
periop	perioperative
PID	pelvic inflammatory disease
pkg	package
pkt	packet
pm	evening
PO	by mouth
postop	postoperative
PR	by rectum
PRC	pregnancy risk category
preop	preoperative
prep	preparation
prev	prevention
prn	as needed
prophx	prophylaxis
PSVT	paroxysmal supraventricular tachycardia
PT	prothrombin time
pt, pts	patient, patients
PTT	partial thromboplastin time
PVC	premature ventricular contraction
pwd	powder
q	every
qid	four times a day
qod	every other day
RA	rheumatoid arthritis
Rad	radiation
RBC	red blood cell
reconst	reconstitute
RNA	ribonucleic acid
RF	renal failure
SC	subcutaneous
sec	second
SL	sublingual
sol	solution
sprink	sprinkles
SSRI	selective serotonin reuptake inhibitor
ST	sinus tachycardia
staph	staphylococci
strep	streptococci
supp	suppository
suppl	supplement
surg	surgery
susp	suspension
sust-rel	sustained-release
SVT	supraventricular tachycardia
syn	syndrome
tab	tablet
TB	tuberculosis
tbl	tablespoon
TCA	tricyclic antidepressant
temp	temperature
tid	three times a day
TMD	target maintenance dose
tsp	teaspoon
tx	treatment
U	unit
URI	upper respiratory infection
UTI	urinary tract infection
vag	vaginal
VF	ventricular fibrillation
VT	ventricular tachycardia
WBC	white bloo cell
wk	week
wkly	weekly
wt	weight
yr	year

Classes	Dosage Forms	Indications & Dosages
abacavir sulfate • Ziagen		
Nucleoside analogue reverse transcriptase inhibitor; antiviral PRC: C	*Oral sol:* 20 mg/ml; *Tab:* 300 mg	*HIV-1 infect*—**Adult:** 300 mg PO bid with other antiretrovirals. **Child 3 mo–16 yr:** 8 mg/kg PO bid (max, 300 mg PO bid) with other antiretrovirals.
acyclovir (acycloguanosine) **acyclovir sodium** • Zovirax		
Synthetic purine nucleoside; antiviral PRC: C	*Caps:* 200 mg; *Inj:* 500 mg/vial, 1 g/vial; *Inj conc for IV inf:* 50 mg/ml; *Oint:* 5%; *Oral susp:* 200 mg/5 ml; *Tab:* 400 mg, 800 mg	*Initial and recurrent mucocutaneous herpes (HSV types 1, 2), severe initial genital herpes, herpes in immunocompromised pts*—**Adult, child ≥ 12 yr:** 5 mg/kg by IV inf at constant rate over 1 h q 8 h × 7 d (5 d genital). **Child < 12 yr:** 10 mg/kg by IV inf at constant rate over 1 h q 8 h × 7 d (5 d genital). *Mucocutaneous herpes (HSV types 1 and 2) in immunocompromised pts*—**Adult:** 400 mg PO q 4 h while awake (5 times/d). **Child:** 1 g PO daily div into three to five doses × 7–14 d. Max, 80 mg/kg/d. *Disseminated herpes zoster*◇—**Adult:** 5 to 10 mg/kg IV q 8 h × 7–10 d. Infuse over ≥ 1 h. *Initial genital herpes*—**Adult:** 200 mg PO q 4 h while awake (5 caps/d) × 10 d. Or, 400 mg PO tid × 7–10 d. *Genital herpes in immunocompromised pts*◇—**Adult:** 400 mg PO 3–5 times/d. *Initial rectal (procitis) herpes infect*◇—**Adult:** 400 mg PO 5 times/d × 10 d or until resolution. Or, 800 mg PO q 8 h × 7–10 d. *Acute herpes zoster*—**Adult:** 800 mg PO 5 times/d × 7–10 d; start within 48 h of rash onset. *Intermittent therapy for recurrent genital herpes*—**Adult:** 200 mg PO q 4 h while awake (5 caps/d) × 5 d. Start at first sign of recurrence.

Long-term suppression of recurrent genital herpes—**Adult:** 400 mg PO bid for up to 1 yr with reevaluation.

Genital herpes; non–life-threatening herpes in immunocompromised pts—**Adult, child:** Cover lesions with oint q 3 h, 6 times/d × 7 d.

Neonatal herpes—**Neonate, infant ≤ 3 mo:** 10 mg/kg IV q 8 h × 10 d. **Preterm neonate:** 10 mg/kg IV q 12 h.

Primary or recurrent herpes in pts with HIV—**Adult:** 200 to 800 mg PO 5 times/d.

Long-term suppression or prophx for recurrent herpes in pts with HIV◇—**Adult, adolescent:** 200 mg PO tid or 400 mg PO bid. **Infant, child:** 600 to 1,000 mg PO daily in three to five div doses. Or, 80 mg/kg in three to four div doses.

Acute varicella (chickenpox) infect—**Adult, child ≥ 2 yr weighing > 40 kg (88 lb):** 800 mg PO qid × 5 d. **Child ≥ 2 yr weighing < 40 kg:** 20 mg/kg PO qid × 5 d.

Acute herpes zoster ophthalmicus◇—**Adult:** 600 mg PO q 4 h 5 times/d × 10 d. Start within 7 d (72 h if possible) of rash onset.

Varicella zoster in immunocompromised pts—**Adult, child ≥ 12 yr:** 10 mg/kg IV over 1 h q 8 h × 7 d. **Child < 12 yr:** 20 mg/kg IV over 1 h q 8 h × 7 d.

HSV encephalitis—**Adult, child > 12 yr:** 10 mg/kg IV over 1 h q 8 h × 10 d. **Infant, child 3 mo–12 yr:** 20 mg/kg q 8 h IV over ≥ 1 h × 10 d.

≡ ***Dosage adjustment.*** If pt receives 200–400 mg PO and CrCl < 10 ml/min, give 200 mg q 12 h. If pt receives 800 mg PO q 4 h 5 times/d, give 800 mg PO q 8 h if CrCl is 10–25 ml/min or q 12 h if < 10 ml/min. Give full IV dose q 12 h if CrCl is 25–50 ml/min or q 24 h if 10–25 ml/min. Give half IV dose q 24 h if CrCl < 10 ml/min.

Classes	Dosage Forms	Indications & Dosages
amantadine hydrochloride • Symmetrel		
Synthetic cyclic primary amine; antiviral, antiparkinsonian PRC: C	*Caps:* 100 mg; *Syrup:* 50 mg/5 ml; *Tab:* 100 mg	*Prophx or tx of influenza type A, respiratory tract illnesses in geriatric or debilitated pts*—**Adult ≤ 64 yr, child ≥ 10 yr weighing > 40 kg (88 lb):** 200 mg/d PO as single dose or div bid. **Child 1–9 yr:** 4.4 to 8.8 mg/kg/d PO (max, 150 mg). To reduce toxicity, 5 mg/kg/d in one to two div doses (max, 150 mg/d). **Adult > 64 yr:** 100 mg PO once/d. Cont 24–48 h after symptoms resolve. Start prophx as soon as possible after exposure and cont ≥ 10 days. May cont 90 d if flu virus vaccine unavailable. If used with vaccine, cont 2–4 wk until protection develops. *Drug-induced extrapyramidal reactions*—**Adult:** 100 to 300 mg/d PO, div. *Idiopathic parkinsonism, parkinsonian syndrome*—**Adult:** 100 mg PO bid; if pt seriously ill or taking other antiparkinsonian drugs, 100 mg daily × ≥ 1 wk; then 100 mg bid, prn. May give up to 400 mg/d, but watch closely if dose > 200 mg. ≡ ***Dosage adjustment.*** If CrCl is 30–50 ml/min, give 200 mg (syrup or caps) d 1 and then 100 mg/d (caps). If 15–29 ml/min, 200 mg d 1 and 100 mg q alternate d. If < 15 ml/min, 200 mg q 7 d. During long-term hemodialysis, 200 mg PO q 7 d.
amikacin sulfate • Amikin		
Aminoglycoside; antibiotic PRC: D	*Inj:* 50 mg/ml, 250 mg/ml	*Serious infect by susceptible organism*—**Adult, child:** 15 mg/kg/d div q 8–12 h over 30–60 min IM or IV (in 100–200 ml D_5W or NSS). Max, 1.5 g/d or 15 mg/kg. **Adult** ◇: 4–20 mg intrathecally or intraventricularly as single dose IM or IV. **Neonate:** 10 mg/kg IM or IV over 1–2 h (in D_5W or NSS); then 7.5 mg/kg q 12 h. *Uncomplicated UTI*—**Adult:** 250 mg IM or IV bid. *Clinical tuberculosis* ◇ —**Adult, child, infant:** 15 mg/kg/d IM, 5 times/wk with

other antituberculotics.

≡ ***Dosage adjustment.*** If renal impairment, 7.5 mg/kg initially; then based on amikacin levels and renal function. May give more 7.5-mg/kg doses at intervals (in h) determined by multiplying steady-state serum creatinine level (in mg/dl) by 9. Keep peak serum level at 15–35 mcg/ml and trough ≤ 5–10 mcg/ml.

amoxicillin trihydrate • Amoxil, Trimox, Wymox

Aminopenicillin; antibiotic
PRC: B

Caps: 250 mg, 500 mg; *Ped drops:* 50 mg/ml (after reconstitution); *Susp:* 125 mg/5 ml, 200 mg/5 ml, 250 mg/5 ml, 400 mg/5 ml; *Tab (chew):* 125 mg, 200 mg, 250 mg, 400 mg; *Tab (film-coated):* 500 mg, 875 mg

Systemic infect, acute or chronic UTI, respiratory tract infect, uncomplicated UTI—**Adult:** 250 mg PO q 8 h or 500 mg q 12 h. Severe infect, up to 500 mg q 8 h or 875 mg q 12 h. **Child:** 20 to 40 mg/kg/d PO, div q 8 h. **Neonate, infant ≤ 12 wk:** 30 mg/kg PO daily in div doses q 12 h. **Child (ped drops):** 0.75 ml q 8 h if < 6 kg (13 lb), 1 ml q 8 h if 6–7 kg (13–15 lb), 1.25 ml q 8 h if 7–8 kg (16–18 lb). **Child with lower respiratory tract infect (ped drops):** 1.25 ml q 8 h if < 6 kg; 1.75 ml q 8 h if 6–7 kg; 2.25 ml q 8 h if 7–8 kg.

Uncomplicated gonorrhea—**Adult:** 3 g PO as single dose. **Child > 2 yr:** 50 mg/kg with 25 mg/kg probenecid as single dose.

Chlamydial and mycoplasmal infect during pregnancy—**Adult:** 500 mg PO tid × 7–10 d.

Lyme disease ◇—**Adult:** 250–500 mg PO tid to qid × 10–30 d. **Child:** 25–50 mg/kg/d (max, 1–2 g/d) PO in three div doses × 10–30 d.

Acute uncomplicated UTI in nonpregnant woman ◇—3 g PO as single dose.

Prophx of bacterial endocarditis—(Consult American Heart Association before giving drug.) **Adult:** 2 g 1 h before procedure. **Child:** 50 mg/kg 1 h before procedure.

Post-exposure prophx to penicillin-susceptible anthrax—**Adult:** 500 mg PO tid × 60 d. **Child:** 80 mg/kg/d PO div into three doses/d × 60 d.

≡ ***Dosage adjustment.*** If CrCl is 10–30 ml/min, incr to q 12 h; if < 10 ml/min, q 24 h. Suppl doses may be needed after hemodialysis. Don't give 875-mg tablet if CrCl < 30 ml/min.

Classes	Dosage Forms	Indications & Dosages
amoxicillin and clavulanate potassium • Augmentin, Augmentin ES-600, Clavulin ◆		
Aminopenicillin and beta-lactamase inhibitor; antibiotic PRC: B	*Oral susp:* 125 mg amoxicillin and 31.25 mg clavulanic acid/5 ml after reconstitution, 200 mg amoxicillin and 28.5 mg clavulanic acid/5 ml, 250 mg amoxicillin and 62.5 mg clavulanic acid/5 ml, 400 mg amoxicillin and 57 mg clavulanic acid/5 ml, 600 mg amoxicillin and 42.9 mg clavulanic acid/5 ml; *Tab:* 250 mg amoxicillin and 125 mg clavulanic acid, 500 mg amoxicillin and 125 mg clavulanic acid, 875 mg amoxicillin and 125 mg clavulanic acid; *Tab (chew):* 125 mg amoxicillin and 31.25 mg clavulanic acid, 200 mg amoxicillin and 28.5 mg clavulanic acid, 250 mg amoxicillin and 62.5 mg clavulanic acid, 400 mg	*Lower respiratory tract infect, OM, sinusitis, skin and skin-structure infect, UTI*—**Adult, child weighing ≥ 40 kg (88 lb):** 250 mg (based on amoxicillin component) PO q 8 h or one 500-mg tablet q 12 h. More severe infect, 500 mg q 8 h or 875 mg q 12 h. **Child weighing < 40 kg:** 25 to 45 mg/kg/d PO (based on amoxicillin) in div doses q 8–12 h. **Neonate, infant < 12 wk:** 30 mg/kg/d div doses q 12 h. *Recurrent or persistent acute otitis media with antibiotic exposure during previous 3 mo in pts ≤ 2 or in daycare, from* Streptococcus pneumoniae, Haemophilus influenzae, Moraxella catarrhalis—**Infant, child 3 mo–12 yr weighing < 40 kg:** 90 mg/kg/d Augmentin ES-600 (based on amoxicillin) PO q 12 h × 10 d. ≡ ***Dosage adjustment.*** If CrCl 15–30 ml/min, usual dose q 12–18 h. If 5–15 ml/min, usual dose q 20–36 h. If < 5 ml/min, usual dose q 48 h. Some advise against drug if < 30 ml/min. During hemodialysis, 500 mg PO midway through tx and 500 mg PO at end of tx.

	amoxicillin and 57 mg clavulanic acid	

amphotericin B • Amphocin, Fungizone

Polyene antibiotic; antifungal PRC: B	*Cream:* 3%; *Lotion:* 3%; *Oint:* 3%; *Oral susp:* 100 mg/ml; *Pwd for inj:* 50 mg	*Systemic (life-threatening) fungal infect, fungal endocarditis, fungal septicemia*—**Adult, child:** Some advise 1 mg IV in 20 ml D_5W over 20 min as initial dose. If tolerated, 0.25–0.30 mg/kg/d, incr by 5–10 mg/d to 1 mg/kg/d or 1.5 mg/kg q alternate d. Duration depends on infect. *Sporotrichosis*—**Adult, child:** 0.4–to 0.5 mg/kg/d amphotericin B IV up to 9 mo. Total IV dosage 2.5 g × 9 mo. *Aspergillosis*—**Adult, child:** 0.5–0.6 mg/kg/d initially. Total IV dosage 1.5–4 g × 11 mo. *Fungal meningitis* ◇—**Adult:** Intrathecal inj of 25 mcg/0.1 ml in 10–20 ml of CSF, given by barbotage 2–3 times/wk. *Candidal cystitis* ◇—**Adult:** Bladder irrigation with 50 mcg/ml periodically or continuously × 5–10 d. *Oropharyngeal candidiasis*—**Adult, child:** 100 mg/ml oral susp qid swish and swallow. *Topical fungal infect (3% cream, lotion, oint)*—**Adult, child:** Apply liberally bid to qid; rub in. *Cutaneous or mucocutaneous candidal infect*—**Adult, child:** Apply bid, tid, or qid × 1–3 wk (up to several mo if interdigital or paronychial). *Sinus irrigation*—**Adult:** 1 mg/ml. *Histoplasmal pulmonary and intrapleural effusion* ◇—**Adult:** 15–20 mg with 25 mg hydrocortisone sodium succinate. *Pulmonary coccidioidomycosis* ◇—**Adult:** 5–10 mg qid via IPPB device. *Ophthalmic candidal infect* ◇—**Adult:** 0.1–1 mg/ml drop susp q 30 min. *Empiric therapy of presumed fungal infect in febrile, neutropenic pt (including cancer, BMT, solid organ transplant pts)*—**Adult:** 0.8 mg/kg/d × 8 d.

Classes	Dosage Forms	Indications & Dosages
amphotericin B cholesteryl sulfate complex • Amphotec		
Polyene antibiotic; antifungal PRC: B	*Inj:* 50 mg/20 ml, 100 mg/50 ml	*Invasive aspergillosis when renal impairment or toxicity precludes conventional amphotericin B, pt with invasive aspergillosis when previous amphotericin B failed;* Candida *and* Cryptococcus *infect when pt unresponsive to or intolerant of amphotericin B* ◇—**Adult, child:** 3–4 mg/kg/d IV by continuous inf at 1 mg/kg/h; may increase to 6 mg/kg/d if no improvement or infect progresses. Before new course, infuse test dose (10 ml of final prep containing 1.6–8.3 mg of drug) over 15–30 min and monitor pt for next 30 min. *Empiric therapy of presumed fungal infect in febrile, neutropenic pt (including cancer, BMT, solid organ transplant pts)* ◇—**Adult:** 4 mg/kg/d IV × 8 d. Up to 7.5 mg/kg have been used to treat invasive fungal infect in BMT.
amphotericin B lipid complex • Abelcet		
Polyene antibiotic; antifungal PRC: B	*Susp for inj:* 100 mg/ 20-ml vial	*Invasive fungal infect (including* Aspergillus *and* Candida *sp.), in pt refractory to or intolerant of conventional amphotericin B*—**Adult, child:** 5 mg/kg/d IV as single inf at 2.5 mg/kg/h.
amphotericin B liposomal • AmBisome		
Polyene antibiotic; antifungal PRC: B	*Inj:* 50-mg vial	*Empiric therapy for fungal infect in febrile, neutropenic pt*—**Adult, child:** 3 mg/kg/d IV inf over 60–120 min. *Systemic fungal infect with* Aspergillus, Candida, *or* Cryptococcus *sp. refractory to amphotericin B; pt in whom renal impairment or toxicity precludes amphotericin B*—**Adult, child:** 3–5 mg/kg/d IV inf over 60–120 min. *Visceral leishmaniasis*—**Immunocompetent adult, child:** 3 mg/kg/d IV inf on d 1–5, 14, and 21. Repeat course may be ordered if initial tx fails to clear parasite. **Immunocompromised adult, child:** 4 mg/kg/d IV inf on d 1–5, 10, 17, 24,

31, and 38. Expert advice needed if initial therapy fails or pt has relapse. *Cryptococcal meningitis in HIV-infected pts*—**Adult, child:** 6 mg/kg/d IV inf over 2 h (1 h if well tolerated, longer if discomfort occurs).

ampicillin • Apo-Ampi ◆, Novo-Ampicillin ◆, Omnipen, Penbritin ◆
ampicillin sodium • Ampicin ◆, Omnipen-N, Penbritin ◆
ampicillin trihydrate • Marcillin, Principen, Totacillin

Aminopenicillin; antibiotic
PRC: B

Caps: 250 mg, 500 mg; *Inf:* 500 mg, 1 g, 2 g; *Parenteral:* 125 mg, 250 mg, 500 mg, 1 g, 2 g; *Susp:* 125 mg/5 ml, 250 mg/5 ml

Systemic infect, acute and chronic UTI—**Adult:** 250–500 mg PO q 6 h. **Child weighing < 40 kg:** 50–100 mg/kg/d PO, div q 6 h; or 100–200 mg/kg/d IV × 3 d and then IM, div q 6–8 h. **Neonate ≤ 1 wk and weighing ≤ 2 kg:** 25 mg/kg IM or IV q 12 h. **Neonate ≤ 1 wk and weighing > 2 kg; neonate > 1 wk and weighing ≤ 2 kg:** 25 mg/kg IM or IV q 8 h. **Neonate > 1 wk and weighing > 2 kg:** 25 mg/kg IM or IV q 6 h.
Meningitis—**Adult:** 8–14 g IV or 150–200 mg/kg/d div q 3–4 h × 3 d; then IM if desired. **Child 2 mo–12 yr:** 200 to 400 mg/kg/d IV div q 4–6 h, maybe with chloramphenicol pending culture results. **Neonate ≤ 1 wk and weighing ≤ 2 kg:** 50–75 mg/kg IV q 12 h. **Neonate ≤ 1 wk and weighing > 2 kg:** 50–75 mg/kg IV q 8 h. **Neonate > 1 wk and weighing ≤ 2 kg:** 50 mg/kg IV q 8 h. **Neonate > 1 wk and weighing > 2 kg:** 50 mg/kg IV q 6 h.
Neonatal group B streptococcal meningitis—**Neonate < 7 days:** 200 mg/kg/d IV in three div doses.
Neonate ≥ 7 days: 300 mg/kg/d IV in four to six div doses.
Uncomplicated gonorrhea—**Adult:** 3.5 g PO with 1 g probenecid as single dose.
≡ ***Dosage adjustment.*** Incr to q 12–16 h in pt with CrCl ≤ 10 ml/min.
Prophx for bacterial endocarditis before dental or minor respiratory procedures—**Adult:** 2 g IV or IM 30 min before procedure. **Child:** 50 mg/kg IV or IM 30 min before procedure.

(continued)

Classes	Dosage Forms	Indications & Dosages
ampicillin **ampicillin sodium** **ampicillin trihydrate** *(continued)*		
		Enterococcal endocarditis—**Adult:** 12 g/d by continuous IV inf or in six equally div doses with gentamicin (1 mg/kg IM or IV q 8 h × 4–6 wk. *Prophx of neonatal group B streptococcus infect* ◇—**Adult:** 2 g IV for mother ≥ 4 h before delivery; then 1–2 g IV q 4–6 h until delivery.
ampicillin sodium and sulbactam sodium • Unasyn		
Aminopenicillin/beta-lactamase inhibitor combination; antibiotic PRC: B	*Inj:* vials and piggyback vials of 1.5 g (1 g ampicillin sodium, 500 mg sulbactam sodium) and 3 g (2 g ampicillin sodium, 1 g sulbactam sodium)	*Skin, skin-structure, intra-abdominal, gyn infect from susceptible gram-pos, gram-neg bacteria, beta-lactamase-producing strains of* Staphylococcus aureus, Escherichia coli, Klebsiella *(including* K. pneumoniae*)*, Proteus mirabilis, Bacteroides *(including* B. fragilis*)*, Enterobacter, Neisseria meningitidis, N. gonorrhoeae, Moraxella catarrhalis, Acinetobacter calcoaceticus—**Adult:** 1.5–3 g IM or IV q 6 h. Max, 4 g/d sulbactam sodium. *Skin, skin-structure infect*—**Child weighing ≥ 40 kg (88 lb):** Adult dose. **Child ≥ 1 yr weighing < 40 kg:** 300 mg/kg/d IV div q 6 h. Max 14 d. ≡ ***Dosage adjustment.*** 1.5–3 g q 6–8 h for CrCl ≥ 30 ml/min, q 12 h for CrCl 15–29 ml/min, q 24 h for CrCl 5–14 ml/min.
amprenavir • Agenerase		
Protease inhibitor; antiretroviral PRC: C	*Caps:* 50 mg, 150 mg; *Oral sol:* 15 mg/ml	*HIV-1 infect (with other antiretrovirals)*—**Adult, adolescent weighing ≥ 50 kg (110 lb):** 1,200 mg PO (8 150-mg caps) bid. **Child 4–12 yr or adolescent weighing < 50 kg:** Caps, 20 mg/kg PO bid or 15 mg/kg PO tid (max, 2,400 mg/d). Oral sol, 22.5 mg/kg PO (1.5 ml/kg) bid or 17 mg/kg PO (1.1 ml/kg) tid (max, 2,800 mg/d).

atovaquone • Mepron

Ubiquinone analogue; antiprotozoal PRC: C	*Susp:* 750 mg/5 ml	*Acute, mild-to-moderate Pneumocystis carinii pneumonia (PCP)*—**Adult, adolescent:** 750 mg PO bid × 21 d with food. **Child** ◇: 40 mg/kg/d PO, two div doses. *Primary and secondary prophx of PCP*—**Adult, adolescent:** 1,500 mg PO once/d with food. **HIV-infected infant 1–3 mo, child > 24 mo** ◇: 30 mg/kg PO once/d. **HIV-infected child 4–24 mo** ◇: 45 mg/kg PO once/d. *Primary prophx of toxoplasmosis in HIV infect* ◇—**Adult, adolescent:** 1,500 mg PO once/d (maybe with pyrimethamine 25 mg once/d or leucovorin 10 mg once/d). **Infant 1–3 mo, child > 24 mo:** 30 mg/kg PO once/d. **Child 4–24 mo:** 45 mg/kg PO once/d. *Prev of recurrence of toxoplasmic encephalitis*—**HIV-infected adult, adolescent:** 750 mg PO q 6–12 h. *Babesiosis* ◇—**Adult:** 750 mg PO bid × 7–10 d (with azithromycin 1 g PO once/d × 3 days; then 500 mg once/d × 7 d). **Child:** 20 mg/kg PO bid × 7–10 d (with azithromycin 12 mg/kg PO once/d × 7–10 d). *Chloroquine-resistant* Plasmodium falciparum *malaria* ◇—**Adult:** 500 mg PO bid × 3 d (with doxycycline 100 mg bid × 3 d). **Child ≥ 8 yr:** 125 (11–20 kg), 250 (21–30 kg), or 375 mg (31–40 kg) PO bid × 3 d (with doxycycline 2 mg/kg/d × 3 d).

atovaquone and proguanil hydrochloride • Malarone

Hydroxynapthalenedione/biguanide hydrochloride; antimalarial PRC: C	*Tab:* 250 mg atovaquone, 100 mg proguanil; 62.5 mg atovaquone, 25 mg proguanil	*Prev of* Plasmodium falciparum *malaria, including areas of chloroquine resistance*—Start 1–2 d before pt enters endemic area and cont until 7 d after return. **Adult, child weighing > 40 kg (88 lb):** One adult-strength tab (250 mg atovaquone, 100 mg proguanil) PO once/d with food or milk. **Child weighing 31–40 kg (68–88 lb):** Three ped-strength tabs PO once/d with food or milk. Total, 187.5 mg atovaquone, 75 mg proguanil daily. *(continued)*

Classes	Dosage Forms	Indications & Dosages
atovaquone and proguanil hydrochloride *(continued)*		
		Child weighing 21–30 kg (46–68 lb): Two ped-strength tabs PO once/d with food or milk. Total, 125 mg atovaquone, 50 mg proguanil daily. **Child weighing 11–20 kg (24–45 lb):** One ped-strength tab/d PO with food or milk. *Tx of acute, uncomplicated* P. falciparum *malaria*—**Adult, child weighing > 40 kg:** Four adult-strength tabs PO once/d × 3 days with food or milk. Total, 1 g atovaquone, 400 mg proguanil daily. **Child weighing 31–40 kg:** Three adult-strength tabs PO once/d × 3 days with food or milk. Total, 750 mg atovaquone, 300 mg proguanil daily. **Child weighing 21–30 kg:** Two adult-strength tabs PO once/d × 3 days with food or milk. Total, 500 mg atovaquone, 200 mg proguanil daily. **Child weighing 11–20 kg:** One adult-strength tab/d × 3 d PO with food or milk.
azelaic acid • Azelex		
Naturally occurring saturated dicarboxylic acid; antiacne drug PRC: B	*Cream:* 20%	*Mild-to-moderate inflammatory acne vulgaris*—**Adult:** Thin film massaged into affected areas am and pm.
azithromycin • Zithromax		
Azalide macrolide; antibiotic PRC: B	*Inj:* 500 mg, *Pwd for oral susp:* 100 mg/5 ml, 200 mg/5 ml, 300 mg ◆, 600 mg ◆, 900 mg ◆, 1,000 mg/packet; *Tab:* 250 mg, 600 mg	*Acute exacer COPD from* Haemophilus influenzae, Moraxella catarrhalis, Streptococcus pneumoniae; *uncomplicated skin and skin-structure infect from* Staphylococcus aureus, Streptococcus pyogenes, Streptococcus agalactiae; *pharyngitis or tonsillitis from* S. pyogenes *(second-line)*—**Adult, adolescent ≥ 16 yr:** 500 mg PO single dose day 1 and 250 mg/d days 2–5. Total, 1.5 g. *Community-acquired pneumonia from* Chlamydia pneumoniae, H. influenzae, Mycoplasma pneumoniae, Streptococcus pneumoniae—**Adult, adolescent**

≥ **16 yr:** 500 mg PO single dose day 1; then 250 mg PO/d days 2–5. Total, 1.5 g. If pt needs initial IV therapy, 500 mg/d IV single dose × 2 d; then 500 mg/d PO single dose to finish 7- to 10-d course. Timing of change from IV to PO based on pt response. IV form can be used for above infect and those caused by *Legionella pneumophila, M. catarrhalis, S. aureus.*

Nongonococcal urethritis or cervicitis from Chlamydia trachomatis—**Adult, adolescent** ≥ **16 yr:** 1 g PO single dose.

Pelvic inflammatory disease from C. trachomatis, Neisseria gonorrhoeae, Mycoplasma hominis *in pts who need initial IV therapy*—**Adult:** 500 mg/d IV single dose × 1–2 d; then 250 mg/d PO to complete 7-day course. Timing of change from IV to PO based on pt response.

Otitis media—**Child > 6 mo:** 30 mg/kg PO single dose, or 10 mg/kg/d PO × 3 d, or 10 mg/kg PO day 1 and 5 mg/kg/d (max, 250 mg) days 2–5.

Tonsillitis—**Child > 2 yr:** 12 mg/kg/d (max, 500 mg) PO × 5 d.

Chancroid—**Adult:** 1 g PO single dose. **Infant, child:** 20 mg/kg (max, 1 g) single dose PO.

Prev of disseminated MAC in pts with advanced HIV infect—**Adult:** 1.2 g/wk PO alone or with rifabutin. **Child:** 20 mg/kg/wk PO (max, 1.2 g) or 5 mg/kg/d (max, 250 mg) PO.

Prophx of bacterial endocarditis in penicillin-allergic adults at moderate-to-high risk—**Adult:** 500 mg 1 h before procedure.

Chlamydial ophthalmia neonatorum ◇—**Infant:** 20 mg/kg PO once/d × 3 d.

aztreonam • Azactam

Monobactam; antibiotic PRC: B	*Inj:* 500-mg, 1-g, 2-g vials	*UTI; respiratory tract, intra-abdominal, gyn, skin infect; septicemia from gram-neg bacteria; adjunct therapy in pelvic inflammatory disease* ◇; *gonorrhea* ◇—**Adult:** 500 mg–2 g IV or IM q 8–12 h. Severe or life-threatening infect: 2 g q 6–8 h. Max, 8 g/d. Gonorrhea: 1 g IM single dose. **Child** ≥ **9 mo:** 30 mg/kg q 6–8 h (depending on severity); up to 120 mg/kg/d. *(continued)*

Classes	Dosage Forms	Indications & Dosages
aztreonam *(continued)*		
		Neonate < 1 wk and weighing ≤ 2 kg: 30 mg/kg IV q 12 h. **Neonate < 1 wk and weighing > 2 kg:** 30 mg/kg IV q 8 h. **Neonate 1–4 wk and weighing ≤ 2 kg:** 30 mg/kg IV q 8 h. **Neonate 1–4 wk and weighing > 2 kg:** 30 mg/kg IV q 6 h. ≡ ***Dosage adjustment.*** In adults with CrCl 10–30 ml/min, half dose after initial dose of 1–2 g. If CrCl < 10 ml/min, initial dose of 500 mg–2 g; then ¼ usual dose at usual intervals and ⅛ initial dose after each hemodialysis session.
bacitracin • AK-Tracin, Altracin, Baciguent, Baci-IM		
Polypeptide antibiotic; antibiotic PRC: C	*Inj:* 50,000-unit vials; *Ophth oint:* 500 units/g; *Topical oint:* 500 units/g (also combination products with neomycin, polymyxin B, bacitracin)	*Topical infect, impetigo, abrasion, cut, minor wound*—**Adult, child:** Thin film to cleansed area 1–3 times/d × ≤ 7 d. *Pneumonia, empyema from staph infect*—**Child weighing ≤ 2.5 kg (5.5 lb):** 900 units/kg/d IM in two to three div doses. **Child weighing > 2.5 kg:** 1,000 units/kg/d IM in two to three div doses. **Adult** ◇: 10,000–25,000 units IM q 6 h. Max, 100,000 units/d. *Antibiotic-related pseudomembranous colitis from* Clostridium difficile ◇—**Adult:** 20,000–25,000 units PO q 6 h × 7–10 d. *Short-term topical tx of superficial infect of conjunctiva and cornea caused by bacitracin-susceptible organisms*—**Adult, child:** Apply ophth oint to affected area once or more/d.
boric acid • Auro-Dri, Dri/Ear, Ear-Dry		
Acidic agent, skin protectant; antibacterial PRC: NR	*Otic sol:* 2.75% boric acid in isopropyl alcohol	*External ear canal infect*—**Adult, child:** 3–8 gtt into ear canal; plug with cotton. Repeat tid or qid.

caspofungin acetate • Cancidas

Glucan synthesis inhibitor; antifungal PRC: C	*Lyophilized pwd for inj:* 50-mg and 70-mg single-use vials	*Invasive aspergillosis in pts refractory to or intolerant of other therapies (amphotericin B, amphotericin B lipid, itraconazole)*—**Adult:** 70-mg loading dose on day 1; then 50 mg/d. Give by slow IV inf over about 1 h. Duration based on severity of underlying disease, recovery from immunosuppression, and response.

cefaclor • Ceclor, Ceclor CD

Second-generation cephalosporin; antibiotic PRC: B	*Caps:* 250 mg, 500 mg; *Susp:* 125 mg/5 ml, 187 mg/5 ml, 250 mg/5 ml, 375 mg/5 ml; *Tab (ext-rel):* 375 mg, 500 mg	*Respiratory tract, urinary tract, skin infect; OM*—**Adult:** 250–500 mg PO q 8 h. For ext-rel tab, 375–500 mg PO q 12 h × 7–10 d. **Child:** 20 mg/kg/d PO (40 mg/kg for severe infect and otitis media) div doses q 8–12 h. Max, 1 g/d. ≡ ***Dosage adjustment.*** Pts receiving hemodialysis or peritoneal dialysis may need dosage adjustment.

cefadroxil • Duricef

First-generation cephalosporin; antibiotic PRC: B	*Caps:* 500 mg; *Susp:* 125 mg/5 ml, 250 mg/5 ml, 500 mg/5 ml; *Tab:* 1 g	*Urinary tract, skin, soft-tissue infect; pharyngitis; tonsillitis*—**Adult:** 1–2 g/d PO, depending on infect. Usually given once or twice/d. **Child:** 30 mg/kg/d PO in two div doses. ≡ ***Dosage adjustment.*** If CrCl 25–50 ml/min, give q 12 h. If CrCl 10–25 ml/min, give q 24 h. If CrCl < 10 ml/min, give q 36 h. Pt receiving hemodialysis may need further dosage adjustment.

cefamandole nafate • Mandol

Second-generation cephalosporin; antibiotic PRC: B	*Inj:* 1 g, 2 g	*Serious respiratory, GU, skin, soft tissue, bone, and joint infect; septicemia; peritonitis*—**Adult:** 500 mg to 1 g IM or IV q 4–8 h. If life-threatening, up to 2 g q 4 h. **Infant, child:** 50–100 mg/kg/d IM or IV in equal div doses q 4–8 h. May incr to 150 mg/kg/d (max is max adult dose) *(continued)*

Classes	Dosage Forms	Indications & Dosages
cefamandole nafate *(continued)*		
		for severe infect. Total daily dose is same for IM and IV and depends on susceptibility of organism and severity of infection. Inject drug deep IM into large muscle mass. ≡ ***Dosage adjustment.*** For severe infect, 1–2 g q 6 h if CrCl > 80 ml/min, 750 mg to 1.5 g q 6 h if CrCl 50–80 ml/min, 750 mg to 1.5 g q 8 h if CrCl 25–50 ml/min, 500 mg to 1 g q 8 h if CrCl 10–25 ml/min, 500–750 mg q 12 h if CrCl 2–10 ml/min, 250–599 mg q 12 h if CrCl < 2 ml/min. For life-threatening infect, 2 g q 4 h if CrCl > 80 ml/min, 1.5 g q 4 h or 2 g q 6 h if CrCl 50–80 ml/min, 1.5 g q 6 h or 2 g q 8 h if CrCl 25–50 ml/min, 1 g q 6 h or 1.25 g q 8 h if CrCl 10–25 ml/min, 670 mg q 8 h or 1 g q 12 h if CrCl 2–10 ml/min, or 500 mg q 8 h or 750 mg q 12 h if CrCl < 2 ml/min.
cefazolin sodium • Ancef, Kefzol		
First-generation cephalosporin; antibiotic PRC: B	*Inj (parenteral):* 250 mg, 500 mg, 1 g, 5 g; *Inf:* 500-mg or 1-g Redi Vials, Faspaks, or ADD-Vantage vials	*Serious respiratory, GU, skin, soft tissue, bone, joint infect; biliary tract infect; septicemia; endocarditis; perioperative prophx; contaminated surgery*◇— **Adult:** 250 mg IM or IV q 8 h to 1 g q 8 h. Max, 12 g/d if life-threatening. **Child > 1 yr:** 25–100 mg/kg/d IM or IV in div doses q 8 h. Total daily dose is same for IM and IV and depends on susceptibility of organism and severity of infect. Inject drug deep IM into large muscle mass. ≡ ***Dosage adjustment.*** For adult, give full dose q 8 h or less if CrCl 35–54 ml/min, half usual dose q 12 h if CrCl 11–34 ml/min, half usual dose q 18–24 h if CrCl ≤ 10 ml/min. For child, give 60% of usual daily dose q 12 h if CrCl 40–70 ml/min, 25% of usual daily dose q 12 h if CrCl 20–40 ml/min, 10% of usual daily dose q 24 h if CrCl 5–20 ml/min. Pt receiving hemodialysis may need further adjustment.

cefdinir • Omnicef

Third-generation cephalosporin; antibiotic
PRC: B

Caps: 300 mg; *Susp:* 125 mg/5 ml

Mild-to-moderate infect from microorganisms causing community-acquired pneumonia, acute exacer of chronic bronchitis, acute maxillary sinusitis, acute bacterial otitis media, uncomplicated skin and skin-structure infect—**Adult, adolescent ≥ 13 yr:** 300 mg PO q 12 h or 600 mg PO q 24 h × 10 d. (Use q-12-h doses for pneumonia and skin infections.) **Child 6 mo–12 yr:** 7 mg/kg PO q 12 h or 14 mg/kg PO q 24 h × 10 d, up to max of 600 mg/d. (Use q-12-h doses for skin infections.)

Pharyngitis, tonsillitis—**Adult, adolescent ≥ 13 yr:** 300 mg PO q 12 h × 5–10 d or 600 mg PO q 24 h × 10 d. **Child 6 mo–12 yr:** 7 mg/kg PO q 12 h × 5–10 d or 14 mg/kg PO q 24 h × 10 d.

≡ ***Dosage adjustment.*** If CrCl < 30 ml/min, reduce dosage to 300 mg PO once/d for adult and 7 mg/kg PO (up to 300 mg) for child. If pt receives long-term hemodialysis, give 300 mg or 7 mg/kg PO at end of each session and then every other d.

cefditoren pivoxil • Spectracef

Semisynthetic third-generation cephalosporin; antibiotic
PRC: B

Tab: 200 mg

Acute bacterial exacer of chronic bronchitis from Haemophilus influenzae, H. parainfluenzae, Streptococcus pneumoniae, Moraxella catarrhalis; *tonsillitis; uncomplicated skin and skin-structure infect*—**Adult, adolescent ≥ 12 yr:** 400 mg PO bid with meals × 10 d.

Pharyngitis or tonsillitis from S. pyogenes—**Adult, adolescent ≥ 12 yr:** 200 mg PO bid with meals × 10 d.

Uncomplicated skin, skin-structure infect from S. pyogenes—**Adult, adolescent ≥ 12 yr:** 200 mg PO bid with meals × 10 d.

≡ ***Dosage adjustment.*** Don't give more than 200 mg bid if CrCl 30–49 ml/min. Give 200 mg/d if CrCl < 30 ml/min.

Classes	Dosage Forms	Indications & Dosages
cefepime hydrochloride • Maxipime		
Semisynthetic third- or fourth-generation cephalosporin; antibiotic PRC: B	*Inj:* 500 mg, 1 g, 2 g	*Mild-to-moderate UTI from* Escherichia coli, Klebsiella pneumoniae, *or* Proteus mirabilis, *including those with concurrent bacteremia*—**Adult:** 500 mg to 1 g IM or IV inf over 30 min q 12 h × 7–10 d. (Use IM route only for infect with *E. coli.*) *Severe UTI including pyelonephritis from* E. coli *or* K. pneumoniae—**Adult:** 2 g IV inf over 30 min q 12 h × 10 d. *Moderate-to-severe pneumonia from* Streptococcus pneumoniae, Pseudomonas aeruginosa, K. pneumoniae, *or* Enterobacter *sp.*—**Adult:** 1–2 g IV inf over 30 min q 12 h × 10 d. *Moderate-to-severe uncomplicated skin and skin-structure infect from* Staphylococcus aureus *(methicillin-susceptible strains) or* Streptococcus pyogenes—**Adult:** 2 g IV inf over 30 min q 12 h × 10 d. *Empiric therapy in febrile neutropenia*—**Adult:** 2 g IV q 8 h × 7 d or until neutropenia resolves. **Child < 40 kg (88 lb):** 50 mg/kg IV q 8 h. *Uncomplicated and complicated UTI; uncomplicated skin, skin-structure infect; pneumonia*—**Child < 40 kg:** 50 mg/kg IV q 12 h. Or, American Academy of Pediatrics recommends for child > 1 mo 1–2 g/d, div bid for mild-to-moderate infect or 2–4 g/d div bid for severe infect. Pediatric dosages shouldn't exceed recommended adult dosages. ≡ ***Dosage adjustment.*** Adjust dosage in renal impairment. Give repeat dose at end of hemodialysis. Give usual dose q 48 h if pt receives continuous ambulatory peritoneal dialysis.
cefixime • Suprax		
Third-generation cephalosporin; antibiotic	*Pwd for oral susp:* 100 mg/5 ml;	*Otitis media; acute bronchitis; acute exacer of chronic bronchitis, pharyngitis, tonsillitis; uncomplicated UTI from* Escherichia coli, Proteus mirabilis; *uncom-*

PRC: B | *Tab:* 200 mg, 400 mg

plicated gonorrhea; disseminated gonococcal infect—**Adult, child > 12 yr or > 50 kg (110 lb):** 400 mg/d PO in one to two div doses; uncomplicated gonorrhea, 400 mg single dose. **Child 6 mo–12 yr and ≤ 50 kg:** 8 mg/kg/d PO in one to two div doses.

≡ ***Dosage adjustment.*** Pts with CrCl < 60 ml/min may need adjustment to prevent toxic levels. If adult's CrCl 21–60 ml/min, give 75% of usual dose. If CrCl ≤ 20 ml/min or pt receives continuous ambulatory peritoneal dialysis, give 50% of usual dose.

cefmetazole sodium • Zefazone

Second-generation cephalosporin; antibiotic
PRC: B

Inj: 1-g vial, 2-g vial, 1 g/50 ml, 2 g/50 ml premixed solution

Lower respiratory tract infect from Streptococcus pneumoniae, Staphylococcus aureus *(penicillinase- and non–penicillinase-producing),* Escherichia coli, Haemophilus influenzae *(non–penicillinase-producing); intra-abdominal infect from* E. coli, Bacteroides fragilis; *skin and skin-structure infect from* S. aureus *(penicillinase- and non–penicillinase-producing),* Staphylococcus epidermidis, Streptococcus pyogenes, Streptococcus agalactiae, E. coli, Proteus mirabilis, Klebsiella pneumoniae, B. fragilis; *UTI from* E. coli—**Adult:** 2 g IV q 6–12 h × 5–14 d.

Prophx for vaginal hysterectomy—**Adult:** 2 g IV single dose 30–90 min before surg or 1 g IV 30–90 min before surg repeated in 8 and 16 h.

Prophx for abdominal hysterectomy—**Adult:** 1 g IV 30–90 min before surg repeated in 8 and 16 h.

Prophx for Cesarean section—**Adult:** After clamping cord, 2 g IV single dose or 1 g IV repeated in 8 and 16 h.

Prophx for colorectal surg—**Adult:** 2 g IV single dose 30–90 min before surg. May follow with 2-g doses in 8 and 16 h.

Prophx for high-risk cholecystectomy—**Adult:** 1 g IV 30–90 min before surg, repeated in 8 and 16 h.

≡ ***Dosage adjustment.*** Give 1–2 g q 12 h if CrCl

(continued)

Classes	Dosage Forms	Indications & Dosages
cefmetazole sodium *(continued)*		
		50–90 ml/min; 1–2 g q 16 h if CrCl is 30–49 ml/min, 1–2 g q 24 h if CrCl is 10–29 ml/min, 1–2 g q 48 h after hemodialysis if CrCl < 10 ml/min.
cefonicid sodium • Monocid		
Second-generation cephalosporin; antibiotic PRC: B	*Inf:* 1 g/100 ml; Inj: 1 g	*Periop prophx in contaminated surg*—**Adult:** 1 g IM or IV 60 min before surg; then 1 g/d IM or IV for 2 d after surg. For Cesarean section, 1 g IM or IV after cord clamped. *Serious infect of lower respiratory tract caused by* Streptococcus pneumoniae, Klebsiella pneumoniae, Escherichia coli, Haemophilus influenzae; *UTI caused by* E. coli, Proteus mirabilis, K. pneumoniae; *skin, skin-structure infect caused by* Staphylococcus aureus, S. epidermidis, Streptococcus pyogenes, Streptococcus agalactiae; *septicemia caused by* S. pneumoniae, E. coli; *bone, joint infect caused by* S. aureus; *preop prophx*—**Adult:** 1 g IV or IM q 24 h; if life-threatening, 2 g q 24 h. ≡ ***Dosage adjustment.*** Give 10–25 mg/kg q 24 h if CrCl 60–79 ml/min, 8–20 mg/kg q 24 h if CrCl 40–59 ml/min, 4–15 mg/kg q 24 h if CrCl 20–39 ml/min, 4–15 mg/kg q 48 h if CrCl 10–19 ml/min, 4–15 mg/kg q 3–5 d if CrCl 5–9 ml/min, 3–4 mg/kg q 3–5 d if CrCl < 5 ml/min.
cefoperazone sodium • Cefobid		
Third-generation cephalosporin; antibiotic PRC: B	*Inf:* 1 g, 2 g piggyback; *Parenteral:* 1 g, 2 g	*Serious respiratory tract, intra-abdominal, gyn, skin, skin-structure, urinary tract, enterococcal infect; bacterial septicemia; periop prophx*◇—**Adult:** 1–2 g q 12 h IM or IV. If severe or caused by less-sensitive organism, may incr to 16 g/d. ≡ ***Dosage adjustment.*** Avoid giving > 1 g/d (base) to adult with renal impairment without serum determinations. If pt receives hemodialysis, give dose afterward.

cefotaxime sodium • Claforan

Third-generation cephalosporin; antibiotic
PRC: B

Inf: 1 g, 2 g; *Inj:* 500 mg, 1 g, 2 g

Serious lower respiratory, urinary, CNS, bone, joint, intra-abdominal, gyn, skin infect; bacteremia; septicemia; pelvic inflammatory disease—**Adult, child ≥ 50 kg (110 lb):** 1 g IV or IM q 6–12 h. Up to 12 g/d if life-threatening. **Child 1 mo–12 yr and < 50 kg:** 50–180 mg/kg/d IV in four or six equal div doses. Higher doses for serious infect (such as meningitis). **Neonate 1–4 wk:** 50 mg/kg IV q 8 h. **Neonate < 1 wk:** 50 mg/kg IV q 12 h. Total dose/d same for IM or IV. Inject deep into large muscle mass.

Uncomplicated gonorrhea—**Adult, adolescent:** 1 g IM single dose.

Periop prophx—**Adult:** 1 g IV or IM 30–90 min before surg.

Disseminated gonococcal infect◇—**Adult:** 1 g IV q 8 h. **Neonate, infant:** 25–50 mg/kg IV or IM q 12 h × 7 d.

Gonococcal ophthalmia◇—**Neonate:** 100 mg IV or IM one dose; may cont until ocular cultures negative at 48–72 h.

Gonorrheal meningitis or arthritis◇—**Neonate, infant:** 25–50 mg/kg IV q 12 h × 10–14 d.

≡ ***Dosage adjustment.*** Adjust dosage in renal impairment. Reduce dosage if CrCl < 20 ml/min to prevent toxic levels.

cefotetan disodium • Cefotan

Second-generation cephalosporin, cephamycin; antibiotic
PRC: B

Inf: 1-g, 2-g piggyback vials; *Frozen, premixed sol:* 1 g, 2 g in 50 ml; *Inj:* 1 g, 2 g

Serious urinary, lower respiratory, gyn, skin, intra-abdominal, bone, joint infect—**Adult:** 500 mg to 3 g IV or IM q 12 h × 5–10 d. Up to 6 g/d if life-threatening. **Child:** 40–60 mg/kg/d IV equal div doses q 12 h.

Periop prophx; contaminated surg◇—**Adult:** 1–2 g IV 30–60 min before surg.

Prophx after Cesarean section—**Adult:** 1–2 g IV as soon as cord clamped. Total dose/d same for IM and IV. Inject deep into large muscle mass.

≡ ***Dosage adjustment.*** Give usual adult dose q 24 h or ½ usual dose q 12 h if CrCl 10–30 ml/min. Give usual adult dose q 48 hours *(continued)*

Classes	Dosage Forms	Indications & Dosages
cefotetan disodium *(continued)*		
		or ¼ usual dose q 12 h if CrCl < 10 ml/min. If pt receives hemodialysis, give ¼ usual adult dose q 24 h on days between sessions and ½ usual dose on d of session.
cefoxitin sodium • Mefoxin		
Second-generation cephalosporin, cephamycin; antibiotic PRC: B	*Inf:* 1 g, 2 g in 50-ml containers; *Inj:* 1 g, 2 g	*Serious respiratory, GU, gyn, skin, soft tissue, bone, joint, blood, intra-abdominal infect*—**Adult:** 1–2 g IV q 6–8 h for uncomplicated infect. Up to 12 g/d if life-threatening. **Child > 3 mo:** 80–160 mg/kg/d IV in four to six equal div doses. Max, 12 g/d. Total daily dose same for IM and IV. Inject deep into large muscle mass. *Periop prophx; contaminated surgery*◇—**Adult:** 2 g IV 30–60 min before surg; then 2 g IV q 6 h × 24 h postop. **Child > 3 mo:** 30–40 mg/kg IV 30–60 min before surg; then 30 mg/kg IV q 6 h × 24 h postop. For contaminated surgery, 1–2 g IV q 6 h with or without IV gentamicin (1.5 mg/kg q 8 h) × 5 d. *Uncomplicated gonorrhea*◇—**Adult:** 2 g IM single dose with 1 g probenecid PO at same time or up to 30 min before. *PID*—**Adult:** 2 g IV q 6 h with doxycycline 100 mg IV or PO q 12 h. (If *Chlamydia trachomatis* suspected, give additional antichlamydial coverage.) ≡ ***Dosage adjustment.*** Give 1–2 g q 8–12 h if CrCl 30–50 ml/min, 1–2 g q 12–24 h if CrCl 10–29 ml/min, 500 mg to 1 g q 12–24 h if CrCl 5–9 ml/min, 500 mg to 1 g q 24–48 h if CrCl < 5 ml/min.
cefpodoxime proxetil • Vantin		
Third-generation cephalosporin; antibiotic	*Oral susp:* 50 mg/5 ml, 100 mg/5 ml; *Tab (film-*	*Acute, community-acquired pneumonia from* Haemophilus influenzae, Streptococcus pneumoniae—**Adult:** 200 mg PO q 12 h × 14 d.

PRC: B	*coated):* 100 mg, 200 mg	*Acute bacterial exacer of chronic bronchitis from non–beta-lactamase-producing strain* H. influenzae, S. pneumoniae, Moraxella catarrhalis—**Adult:** 200 mg PO q 12 h × 10 d. *Uncomplicated gonorrhea; rectal gonococcal infect in women*—**Adult:** 200 mg PO single dose. Follow with doxycycline 100 mg PO bid × 7 d. *Uncomplicated skin, skin-structure infect from* Staphylococcus aureus, Streptococcus pyogenes—**Adult:** 400 mg PO q 12 h × 7–14 d. *Acute otitis media from* S. pneumoniae, H. influenzae, M. catarrhalis—**Child 2 mo–12 yr:** 5 mg/kg (max, 200 mg) PO q 12 h × 5 d. *Pharyngitis, tonsillitis from* S. pyogenes—**Adult:** 100 mg PO q 12 h × 7–10 d. **Child 2 mo–12 yr:** 5 mg/kg (max, 100 mg) PO q 12 h × 5–10 d. *Uncomplicated UTI from* Escherichia coli, Klebsiella pneumoniae, Proteus mirabilis, Staphylococcus saprophyticus—**Adult:** 100 mg PO q 12 h × 7 d. *Acute maxillary sinusitis*—**Child 2 mo–12 yr:** 5 mg/kg (max, 200 mg) q 12 h × 10 d. ≡ ***Dosage adjustment.*** Incr interval to q 24 h if CrCl < 30 ml/min. If pt receives hemodialysis, give drug three times/wk, after session.

cefprozil • Cefzil

Second-generation cephalosporin; antibiotic PRC: B	*Oral susp:* 125 mg/5 ml, 250 mg/5 ml; *Tab:* 250 mg, 500 mg	*Pharyngitis or tonsillitis from* Streptococcus pyogenes—**Adult, child ≥ 13 yr:** 500 mg/d PO × ≥ 10 d. **Child 2–12 yr:** 7.5 mg/kg PO q 12 h × 10 d. *Otitis media from* Streptococcus pneumoniae, Haemophilus influenzae, Moraxella catarrhalis—**Infant, child 6 mo–12 yr:** 15 mg/kg PO q 12 h × 10 d. *Secondary bacterial infect of acute bronchitis and acute bacterial exacer of chronic bronchitis from* S. pneumoniae, H. influenzae, M. catarrhalis—**Adult:** 500 mg PO q 12 h × 10 d. *Uncomplicated skin, skin-structure infect from* Staphylococcus aureus *or* S. pyogenes—**Adult, child ≥ 13 yr:** 250 mg PO bid or *(continued)*

Classes	Dosage Forms	Indications & Dosages
cefprozil *(continued)*		
		500 mg once/d or bid × 10 d. **Child 2–12 yr:** 20 mg/kg PO q 24 h × 10 d. ≡ ***Dosage adjustment.*** For CrCl ≤ 30 ml/min, reduce dose by half but maintain interval. Drug is partly removed by hemodialysis; give dose after session.
ceftazidime • Ceptaz, Fortaz, Tazicef, Tazidime		
Third-generation cephalosporin; antibiotic PRC: B	*Inf:* 1 g, 2 g in 50- and 100-ml vials and bags; *Inj:* 500 mg, 1 g, 2 g	*Bacteremia; septicemia; serious respiratory tract, urinary tract, gyn, bone, joint, intra-abdominal, CNS, skin infect*—**Adult:** 1 g IV or IM q 8–12 h; up to 6 g/d if life-threatening. **Child 1 mo–12 yr:** 25–50 mg/kg IV q 8 h. Max, 6 g/d (Fortaz, Tazicef, Tazidime). **Neonate ≤ 4 wk:** 30 mg/kg IV q 12 h (Fortaz, Tazicef, Tazidime). Total dose/d same for IM or IV. Inject deep into large muscle mass. *Empiric therapy in febrile neutropenic pts* ◇—**Adult:** 100 mg/kg/d IV three div doses or 2 g IV q 8 h alone or with an aminoglycoside such as amikacin. **Child ≥ 2 yr:** 50 mg/kg (max, 2 g) q 8 h IV. ≡ ***Dosage adjustment.*** If CrCl ≤ 50 ml/minute, give 1-g loading dose and following maintenance doses. If CrCl 31–50 ml/min, give 1 g q 12 h. If CrCl 16–30 ml/min, give 1 g q 24 h. If CrCl 6–15 ml/min, give 500 mg q 24 h. If CrCl ≤ 5 ml/min, give 500 mg q 48 h. Give 1 g after each hemodialysis session or 500 mg q 24 h if pt receives peritoneal dialysis.
ceftizoxime sodium • Cefizox		
Third-generation cephalosporin; antibiotic PRC: B	*Inf:* 1 g, 2 g in 100-ml vials; *Inj:* 500 mg, 1 g, 2 g	*Bacteremia; septicemia; meningitis; pelvic inflammatory disease; serious respiratory tract, urinary tract, gyn, intra-abdominal, bone, joint, skin infect*—**Adult:** 500 mg to 2 g IV or IM q 8–12 h. If life-threatening, 3–4 g IV q 8 h. **Child ≥ 6 mo:** 50 mg/kg IV or IM q 6–8 h, to 200 mg/kg/d. Total dose/d same for IM or IV. Inject deep into large muscle mass.

Uncomplicated gonorrhea—Adult: 1 g IM single dose.
≡ ***Dosage adjustment.*** For less severe infect, give 500 mg q 8 h if CrCl 50–79 ml/min, 250–500 mg q 12 h if CrCl 5–49 ml/min, and 500 mg q 48 h or 250 mg q 24 h if CrCl < 4 ml/min. For life-threatening infect, give 750 mg to 1.5 g q 8 h if CrCl 50–79 ml/min, 500 mg to 1 g q 12 h if CrCl 5–49 ml/min, and 500 mg to 1 g q 48 h or 500 mg q 24 h if CrCl < 4 ml/min.

ceftriaxone sodium • Rocephin

Third-generation cephalosporin; antibiotic
PRC : B

Inf: 1 g, 2 g; *Inj:* 250 mg, 500 mg, 1 g, 2 g

Bacteremia; septicemia; serious respiratory tract, bone, joint, urinary tract, gyn, intra-abdominal, skin infect—**Adult, child ≥ 12 yr:** 1–2 g IM or IV once/d or in equal div doses bid. Max, 4 g/d. **Child < 12 yr:** 50 to 75 mg/kg/d IM or IV in div doses q 12 h. Max, 2 g/d.
Gonococcal meningitis, endocarditis ◇—**Adult:** 1–2 g IV q 12 h × 10–14 d (meningitis) or 3–4 wk (endocarditis). **Child:** 50–100 mg/kg (max, 4 g/d) IM or IV once/d or div q 12 h × 7–14 d (meningitis) or 28 d (endocarditis). May give initial 100-mg/kg dose (max, 4 g) IM or IV to start. Total dose/d same for IM or IV. Inject deep into large muscle mass.
Preop prophx—**Adult:** 1 g IM or IV 30 min to 2 h before surg.
Uncomplicated gonorrhea—**Adult:** 125–250 mg IM single dose.
Haemophilus ducreyi *infect* ◇—**Adult:** 250 mg IM single dose.
Sexually transmitted epididymitis ◇—**Adult:** 250 mg IM single dose, followed by other antibiotics.
Pelvic inflammatory disease—**Adult:** 250 mg IM single dose, followed by doxycycline 100 mg PO bid × 14 d.
Anti-infective for sexual assault victim ◇—**Adult:** 125 mg IM single dose with other antibiotics.
Lyme disease ◇—**Adult:** 2 g IV q 12–24 h × 14–28 d. **Child:** 75–100 mg/kg IM or IV once/d × 14–28 d.

(continued)

Classes	Dosage Forms	Indications & Dosages
ceftriaxone sodium *(continued)*		
		Persisting or relapsing OM◇—**Child ≥ 3 mo:** 50 mg/kg IM once/d × 3 d. ≡ ***Dosage adjustment.*** If renal impairment, don't exceed 2 g/d without monitoring serum levels.
cefuroxime axetil • Ceftin **cefuroxime sodium** • Kefurox, Zinacef		
Second-generation cephalosporin; antibiotic PRC: B	**cefuroxime axetil** *Susp:* 125 mg/5 ml, 250 mg/5 ml; *Tab (film-coated):* 125 mg, 250 mg, 500 mg **cefuroxime sodium** *Inf:* 750-mg, 1.5-g inf packets; *Inj:* 750 mg, 1.5 g	*Serious lower respiratory, urinary tract, skin, skin-structure infect; septicemia; meningitis*—**Adult:** 750 mg to 1.5 g IM or IV q 8 h × 5–10 d. If life-threatening or caused by less susceptible organism, 1.5 g IM or IV q 6 h. For bacterial meningitis, up to 3 g IV q 8 h. **Child, infant > 3 mo:** 50–100 mg/kg/d IM or IV div doses q 6–8 h. Some give 100–150 mg/kg/d. Meningitis: 200–240 mg/kg/d IV div doses q 6–8 h, reduced to 100 mg/kg/d when pt improves. Some prefer other drugs for meningitis. *Pharyngitis, tonsillitis, lower respiratory tract infect, UTI*—**Adult, child > 12 yr:** 125–500 mg PO bid × 10 d. **Child < 12 yr who can swallow pills:** 125–250 mg PO bid (tab) × 10 d. **Infant, child 3 mo–12 yr:** 20 mg/kg/d PO div doses bid (oral susp) to max of 500 mg × 10 d. *Otitis media, impetigo*—**Infant, child 3 mo–12 yr:** 30 mg/kg/d PO oral susp in two div doses (max dose, 1 g) × 10 d, or 250 mg (tab) PO bid × 10 d. *Periop prophx*—**Adult:** 1.5 g IV 30–60 min before surg; then 750 mg IM or IV q 8 h intraop for prolonged procedure. Open-heart surg pts can receive 1.5 g IV at induction, then q 12 h for three doses. *Gonorrhea (urethral, endocervical, rectal)*—**Adult:** 1.5 g IM single dose, alone or with other antibiotics.

Lyme disease (erythema migrans) from Borrelia burgdoferi—**Adult, adolescent ≥ 13 yr:** 500 mg PO bid × 20 d.

≡ ***Dosage adjustment.*** Safety in renal impairment not known. If CrCl 10–20 ml/min, give 750 mg q 12 h. If CrCl < 10 ml/min, give 750 mg q 24 h. If pt receives hemodialysis, give additional 750 mg at end of each session.

cephalexin hydrochloride • Keftab
cephalexin monohydrate • Biocef, Keflex, Novo-Lexin ◆

First-generation cephalosporin; antibiotic
PRC: B

cephalexin hydrochloride *Tab:* 500 mg; **cephalexin monohydrate** *Caps:* 250 mg, 500 mg; *Susp:* 125 mg/5 ml, 250 mg/5 ml; *Tab (film-coated):* 250 mg, 500 mg, 1g

Respiratory tract, GU tract, skin, soft tissue, bone, joint infect—**Adult:** 250 mg to 1 g PO q 6 h. **Child:** 25–50 mg/kg/d PO in four div doses. In pts > 1 yr with streptococcal pharyngitis or skin or skin-structure infect, daily dose may be two equal div doses q 12 h.

Otitis media—**Adult:** 250 mg to 1 g PO q 6 h. **Child:** 75–100 mg/kg/d PO in four div doses.

≡ ***Dosage adjustment.*** If CrCl 11–40 ml/min, give 500 mg q 8–12 h (adult pt). If CrCl 5–10 ml/min, give 250 mg q 12 h. If CrCl < 5 ml/min, give 250 mg q 12–24 h.

cephradine • Velosef

First-generation cephalosporin; antibiotic
PRC: B

Caps: 250 mg, 500 mg; *Susp:* 125 mg/5 ml, 250 mg/5 ml

Serious respiratory tract, GU tract, skin, soft tissue, bone, joint infect; septicemia; endocarditis; otitis media—**Adult:** 250–500 mg PO q 6 h or 500 mg PO q 12 h. Severe or chronic infect may need larger or more frequent doses (up to 1 g PO q 6 h). **Child > 9 mo:** 25–100 mg/kg/d PO equal div doses q 6–12 h.

≡ ***Dosage adjustment.*** If CrCl 5–20 ml/min, give 250 mg q 6 h. If CrCl < 5 ml/min, give 250 mg q 12 h. If pt receives long-term intermittent dialysis, give 250 mg initially; repeat in 12 h and after 36–48 h. Child's dose may need adjustment based on weight and severity of infection.

Classes	Dosage Forms	Indications & Dosages
chloramphenicol • AK-Chlor, Chloromycetin, Chloroptic, Fenicol ◆, Ocu-Chlor, Pentamycetin ◆ **chloramphenicol sodium succinate** • Chloromycetin Sodium Succinate, Pentamycetin ◆		
Dichloroacetic acid derivative; antibiotic PRC: C	*Inj:* 1-g vial; *Ophth oint:* 1%; *Ophth sol:* 0.5%; *Otic sol:* 0.5%; *Pwd for sol:* 25 mg/vial	*Severe meningitis, brain abscess, bacteremia, other serious infect*—**Adult, child:** 50–100 mg/kg/d IV, div q 6 h. Max, 100 mg/kg/d. **Premature infant, neonate < 7 d or weighing < 2 kg (4.4 lb):** 25 mg/kg/d IV. **Neonate ≥ 7 d and weighing > 2 kg:** 25 mg/kg IV q 12 h. IV route must be used to treat meningitis. *Superficial skin infect*—**Adult, child:** Rub in bid or tid. *External ear canal infect*—**Adult, child:** 2–3 gtt in ear canal tid or qid. *Surface bacterial infect of conjunctiva or cornea*—**Adult, child:** 2 gtt q h until condition improves. Or qid depending on severity. Apply small amt oint to lower conjunctival sac hs to suppl gtt. To use oint alone, apply small amt to lower conjunctival sac q 3–6 h or more often if needed. Cont tx up to 48 h after condition improves.
chloroquine hydrochloride • Aralen Hydrochloride **chloroquine phosphate** • Aralen Phosphate		
4-aminoquinoline; antimalarial, amebicide, anti-inflammatory PRC: C	**chloroquine hydrochloride** *Inj:* 50 mg/ml (40 mg/ml base); **chloroquine phosphate** *Tab:* 500 mg (300-mg base), 250 mg (150-mg base)	*Suppressive prophx*—**Adult:** 500 mg (300-mg base) PO on same d once/wk starting 2 wk before exposure. **Child:** 5 mg (base)/kg PO on same d once/wk (max, adult dosage) starting 2 wk before exposure. *Acute malaria attacks*—**Adult:** 1 g (600-mg base) PO; then 500 mg (300-mg base) PO after 6–8 h; then 500 mg (300-mg base) single dose PO for next 2 d. Or, 4–5 ml (160- to 200-mg base) IM repeated in 6 h if needed. Change to PO ASAP. **Child:** 10 mg (base)/kg PO; then 5 mg (base)/kg after 6 h; then 5 mg (base)/kg 18 h after second dose; then 5 mg (base)/kg 24 h after third dose. Or, 5 mg (base)/kg IM, repeated in 6 h; change to PO ASAP.

Extraintestinal amebiasis—**Adult:** 1 g/d (600-mg base) × 2 d; then 500 mg/d (300-mg base) × 2–3 wk or 4–5 ml (160- to 200-mg base) IM × 10–12 d. Change to PO ASAP. Give with intestinal amebicide.
Rheumatoid arthritis ◇—**Adult:** 250 mg/d PO (chloroquine phosphate) with evening meal.
Lupus erythematosus ◇—**Adult:** 250 mg/d PO (chloroquine phosphate) with evening meal; reduce gradually over several mo when lesions regress.

cidofovir • Vistide

Nucleotide analogue; antiviral
PRC: C

Inj: 75 mg/ml

CMV retinitis in pts with AIDS; acyclovir-resistant HSV infect in immunocompromised pts ◇—**Adult:** 5 mg/kg IV inf over 1 h once/wk × 2 wk followed by maint of 5 mg/kg IV inf over 1 h once q 2 wk. Given with probenecid.
≡ ***Dosage adjustment.*** Start therapy only if creatinine level ≤ 1.5 mg/dl, calculated CrCl > 55 ml/min, and urine protein level < 100 mg/dl (+2 proteinuria). After therapy starts, if creatinine level incr by 0.3–0.4 mg/dl above baseline, reduce dosage to 3 mg/kg. Stop drug if creatinine incr by ≥ 0.5 mg/dl above baseline or +3 proteinuria develops.

ciprofloxacin (systemic) • Cipro

Fluoroquinolone; antibiotic
PRC: C

Inj: 200 mg, 400 mg; *Oral susp:* 250 mg/5 ml, 500 mg/5 ml; *Tab (film-coated):* 100 mg, 250 mg, 500 mg, 750 mg

Mild-to-moderate UTI—**Adult:** 250 mg PO or 200 mg IV q 12 h.
Infectious diarrhea; mild-to-moderate respiratory tract infect; bone, joint infect; severe or complicated UTI—**Adult:** 500 mg PO q 12 h or 400 mg IV q 12 h.
Severe or complicated respiratory tract infect, bone, joint, skin, skin-structure infect; mycobacterial infect—**Adult:** 750 mg PO q 12 h or 400 mg IV q 12 h.
Typhoid fever—**Adult:** 500 mg PO q 12 h.
Intra-abdominal infect (with metronidazole)—**Adult:** 500 mg PO q 12 h or 400 mg IV q 12 h.
Mild-to-moderate acute sinusitis from Haemophilus *(continued)*

Classes	Dosage Forms	Indications & Dosages
ciprofloxacin (systemic) *(continued)*		
		influenzae, Streptococcus pneumoniae, Moraxella catarrhalis; *mild-to-moderate chronic bacterial prostatitis from* Escherichia coli, Proteus mirabilis—**Adult:** 400 mg IV inf over 60 min q 12 h or 500 mg PO q 12 h. *Uncomplicated gonorrhea*—**Adult:** 250 mg PO single dose. *Neisseria meningitidis in nasal passages* ◇—**Adult:** 500–750 mg PO single dose, or 250 mg PO bid × 2 d, or 500 mg PO bid × 5 d. *Inhal anthrax (post-exposure)*—**Adult:** 400 mg q 12 h IV until susceptibility known; then 500 mg PO bid. **Child:** 10 mg/kg q 12 h IV; then 15 mg/kg PO q 12 h. Max, 800 mg/d IV or 1,000 mg/d PO. All pts should receive one or two additional antimicrobials. Switch to PO when appropriate. Treat × 60 d (IV and PO combined). *Cutaneous anthrax* ◇—**Adult:** 500 mg PO bid × 60 d. **Child:** 10–15 mg/kg q 12 h. Max, 1,000 mg/d. Treat × 60 d. ≡ ***Dosage adjustment.*** If adult's CrCl 30–50 ml/min, give 250–500 mg PO q 12 h. If CrCl 5–29 ml/min, give 250–500 mg PO q 18 h or 200–400 mg IV q 18–24 h. If pt receiving hemodialysis or peritoneal dialysis, give 250–500 mg PO q 24 h (after session). Or, for hemodialysis, give 200–400 mg IV q 24 h (after session).
ciprofloxacin hydrochloride (ophthalmic) • Ciloxan		
Fluoroquinolone; antibiotic PRC: C	*Ophth sol:* 0.3% in 2.5- and 5-ml containers	*Corneal ulcers from* Pseudomonas aeruginosa, Staphylococcus aureus, Staphylococcus epidermidis, Streptococcus pneumoniae, *and possibly* Serratia marcescens *and* Streptococcus viridans—**Adult, child > 12 yr:** 2 gtt in affected eye q 15 min × first 6 h; then 2 gtt q 30 min for remainder of d 1. On d 2, give 2 gtt q h. On d 3–14, give 2 gtt q 4 h. *Bacterial conjunctivitis from* S. aureus, S. epidermidis, *possibly* S. pneu-

moniae—**Adult, child > 12 yr:** 1–2 gtt into conjunctival sac of affected eye q 2 h while awake × first 2 d. Then 1–2 gtt q 4 h while awake × next 5 d.

clarithromycin • Biaxin, Biaxin XL

Macrolide; antibiotic PRC: C	*Susp:* 125 mg/5 ml, 250 mg/5 ml, 187 mg/5 ml; *Tab:* 250 mg, 500 mg; *Tab (ext-rel):* 500 mg	*Pharyngitis or tonsillitis from* Streptococcus pyogenes—**Adult:** 250 mg PO q 12 h × 10 d. **Child:** 15 mg/kg/d PO div q 12 h × 10 d. *Acute maxillary sinusitis from* Streptococcus pneumoniae, Haemophilus influenzae, Moraxella catarrhalis—**Adult:** 500 mg PO q 12 h × 14 d. Or, two 500-mg tab (ext-rel) PO once/d × 14 d. **Child:** 15 mg/kg/d PO div q 12 h × 10 d. *Acute exacer of chronic bronchitis from* M. catarrhalis *or* S. pneumoniae; *pneumonia from* S. pneumoniae, Mycoplasma pneumoniae, H. influenzae—**Adult:** 250 mg PO q 12 h × 7–14 d. Or, two 500-mg tab (ext-rel) PO once/d × 7 d. *Acute exacer of chronic bronchitis from* H. influenzae—**Adult:** 500 mg PO q 12 h × 7–14 d. Or, two 500-mg tab (ext-rel) PO once/d × 7 d. *Uncomplicated skin, skin-structure infect from* Staphylococcus aureus, S. pyogenes—**Adult:** 250 mg PO q 12 h × 7–14 d. *Prophx, tx of disseminated infect from MAC*—**Adult:** 500 mg PO bid. **Child:** 7.5 mg/kg PO bid (to 500 mg bid). *Acute otitis media from* H. influenzae, M. catarrhalis, S. pneumoniae—**Child:** 7.5 mg/kg PO bid (to 500 mg bid). Helicobacter pylori *eradication to reduce risk of duodenal ulcer recurrence*—**Adult:** 500 mg Biaxin with 30 mg lansoprazole and 1 g amoxicilin, all given q 12 h × 10–14 d. Or, 500 mg Biaxin q 8 h and 40 mg omeprazole once/d × 14 d. Or, 500 mg Biaxin q 8 h and 400 mg ranitidine bismuth citrate q 12 h × 14 d. *Community-acquired pneumonia from* Chlamydia pneumoniae, M. pneumoniae, S. pneumoniae, H. influenzae—**Adult:** 250 mg PO q 12 h × 7–14 d.

(continued)

Classes	Dosage Forms	Indications & Dosages
clarithromycin *(continued)*		
		Mild-to-moderate community-acquired pneumonia from H. influenzae, H. parainfluenzae, M catarrhalis, S. pneumoniae, C. pneumoniae, M. pneumoniae—**Adult:** two 500-mg tab (ext-rel) PO once/d × 7 d. ≡ ***Dosage adjustment.*** If CrCl < 30 ml/min, reduce dose by half or double the dosing interval.
clindamycin hydrochloride • Cleocin **clindamycin palmitate hydrochloride** • Cleocin Pediatric **clindamycin phosphate** • Cleocin Phosphate, Cleocin T		
Lincomycin derivative; antibiotic PRC: B	*Caps:* 75 mg, 150 mg, 300 mg; *Gel, lotion, pledgets, topical sol:* 1%; *Inf:* 150 mg/ml; *Inj:* 150 mg/ml; *Sol (granules):* 75 mg/5 ml; *Vaginal cream:* 2%	*Infect*—**Adult:** 150–450 mg PO q 6 h. Or, 600–2,700 mg/d IM or IV in two to four equal div doses. Max, 4.8 g/d. **Infant, child > 1 mo:** 8–20 mg/kg/d PO or 20–40 mg/kg/d IV in three to four equal div doses. **Neonate ≤ 1 mo:** 15–20 mg/kg/d IV in three to four equal div doses. *Bacterial vaginosis*—**Adult:** 100 mg (one applicatorful clindamycin phosphate) vaginally hs × 7 d. *Acne vulgaris*—**Adult:** Thin film topical sol, gel, pledget, or lotion to affected area bid. *Toxoplasmosis (cerebral or ocular) in immunocompromised pts*◇—**Adult, adolescent:** 300–450 mg PO q 6–8 h with pyrimethamine (25–75 mg once/d) and leucovorin (10–25 mg once/d). **Infant, child:** 20–30 mg/kg/d PO in four div doses with pyrimethamine (1 mg/kg/d PO) and leucovorin (5 mg once q 3 d PO). Pneumocystis carinii *pneumonia*◇—**Adult:** 600 mg IV q 6 h or 300–450 mg PO qid. With primaquine, give 15–30 mg/d PO.

clofazimine • Lamprene

Substituted iminophenazine dye; leprostatic PRC: C	*Caps:* 50 mg	*Dapsone-sensitive multibacillary leprosy*—**Adult:** 50 mg PO once/d with additional 300 mg PO once/mo combined with two other drugs for 12 mo. *Dapsone-resistant leprosy*—**Adult:** 100 mg PO once/d, usually with one or more other antileprotics × ≥ 3 yr; then monotherapy at 100 mg/d. *Erythema nodosum leprosum*—**Adult:** 100–200 mg/d PO × up to 3 mo. Taper to 100 mg/d ASAP. More than 200 mg/d not recommended. *Atypical mycobacterial infect*◇—**Adult:** 100 mg PO q 8 h. Usually given with several other antituberculotics.

clotrimazole • FemCare, Gyne-Lotrimin 3, Lotrimin, Lotrimin AF, Mycelex-7

Synthetic imidazole derivative; topical antifungal PRC: B (C, oral form)	*Lozenges:* 10 mg; *Cream:* 1%; Lotion: 1%; *Topical sol:* 1%; *Vaginal supp:* 100 mg, 200 mg, 500 mg *Combination pack:* Vaginal supp 100 mg/topical cream 1% 7 g, 200 mg/topical cream 1% 7 g, 500 mg/topical cream 1% 7 g; *Vaginal cream:* 1%, 2%	*Tinea pedis, cruris, versicolor, corporis; cutaneous candidiasis*—**Adult, child:** Massage thin layer into clean affected and surrounding area, morning and evening, usually × 1–4 wk; however, tx may last up to 8 wk. *Vulvovaginal candidiasis*—**Adult:** One supp (100 mg) vaginally hs × 7 d. Or, one supp (200 mg) vaginally × 3 d. For cream, insert one applicatorful vaginally hs × 3–7 d. *Oropharyngeal candidiasis*—**Adult, child:** One lozenge PO 5 times/d × 14 d. *Prophx of oropharyngeal candidiasis in immunocompromised pts*—**Adult:** One lozenge tid throughout chemotherapy. *Keratitis*◇—**Adult:** 1% oint in sterile peanut oil q 2–4 h up to 6 wk.

cloxacillin sodium • Cloxapen

Penicillinase-resistant penicillin; antibiotic PRC: B	*Caps:* 250 mg, 500 mg; *Oral sol:* 125 mg/5 ml (after reconst)	*Systemic infect from penicillinase-producing staphylococci*—**Adult:** 250–500 mg PO q 6 h. **Child:** 50–100 mg/kg/d PO, div and given q 6 h.

Classes	Dosage Forms	Indications & Dosages
co-trimoxazole (trimethoprim-sulfamethoxazole) • Apo-Sulfatrim ♦, Bactrim, Bactrim DS, Bactrim I.V., Cotrim, Cotrim D.S., Novo-Trimel ♦, Roubac ♦, Septra, Septra DS, Septra I.V., SMZ-TMP, Sulfatrim		
Sulfonamide and folate antagonist; antibiotic PRC: C	*Inj:* trimethoprim 16 mg/ml and sulfamethoxazole 80 mg/ml; *Susp:* trimethoprim 40 mg and sulfamethoxazole 200 mg/5 ml; *Tab:* trimethoprim 80 mg and sulfamethoxazole 400 mg; trimethoprim 160 mg and sulfamethoxazole 800 mg	*UTI, shigellosis*—**Adult:** One double-strength or two regular-strength tab PO q 12 h × 10–14 d (5 d shigellosis). Or, 8–10 mg/kg/d (based on trimethoprim) IV in two to four equal div doses up to 14 d (5 d shigellosis). Max, 960 mg/d. **Child, infant ≥ 2 mo:** 8 mg/kg/d trimethoprim and 40 mg/kg/d sulfamethoxazole PO in two div doses q 12 h (10 d UTI; 5 d shigellosis). *Primary prophx for toxoplasmosis in HIV-infected pts*—**Adult, adolescent:** 160 mg/d (based on trimethoprim) PO. **Child:** 150 mg/m²/d (based on trimethoprim) PO in two div doses. *Otitis media*—**Child, infant ≥ 2 mo:** 8 mg/kg/d trimethoprim and 40 mg/kg/d sulfamethoxazole PO in two div doses q 12 h × 10 d. Pneumocystis carinii *pneumonitis*—**Adult, child, infant ≥ 2 mo:** 15–20 mg/kg/d trimethoprim and 75–100 mg/kg/d sulfamethoxazole PO in equal div doses q 6–8 h × 14–21 d. *Prophx of* P. carinii *pneumonia*—**Adult:** 160 mg/d (based on trimethoprim). **Child:** 150 mg/m²/d (based on trimethoprim) in two div doses × 3 d/wk. *Chronic bronchitis*—**Adult:** One double-strength or two regular-strength tab PO q 12 h × 14 d. *Traveler's diarrhea*—**Adult:** One double-strength or two regular-strength tab PO q 12 h × 5 d. Note: For the following off-label uses, dosages refer to oral trimethoprim (as cotrimoxazole). *Septic agranulocytosis* ◇—**Adult:** 2.5 mg/kg IV qid; for prophyx, 80–160 mg bid. *Nocardia infect* ◇—**Adult:** 640 mg/d PO × 7 mo.

Pharyngeal gonococcal infect ◇—**Adult:** 720 mg/d PO × 5 d.
Chancroid ◇—**Adult:** 160 mg PO bid × 7 d.
Pertussis ◇—**Adult:** 320 mg/d PO in two div doses. Child: 40 mg/kg/d PO in two div doses.
Cholera ◇—**Adult:** 160 mg PO bid × 3 d. Child: 5 mg/kg PO bid × 3 d.
Isosporiasis ◇—**Adult:** 160 mg PO qid × 10 d, followed by 160 mg bid × 3 wk.
≡ ***Dosage adjustment.*** If CrCl 15–30 mg/min, give half usual regimen. If CrCl < 15 ml/min, use isn't recommended.

cycloserine • Seromycin

Isoxizolidone, d-alanine analogue; antitubercu-lotic
PRC: C

Caps: 250 mg

Adjunct tx in pulmonary or extrapulmonary TB—**Adult:** 250 mg PO q 12 h × 2 wk; then, if blood level < 25–30 mcg/ml and no signs of toxicity, incr dosage to 250 mg PO q 8 h × 2 wk. If level still not optimum and no signs of toxicity, incr dosage to 250 mg PO q 6 h. Max, 1 g/d. If CNS toxicity occurs, stop drug for 1 wk; then resume at 250 mg/d × 2 wk. If no serious toxic effects, incr dosage by 250-mg steps q 10 d until level reaches 25–30 mcg/ml. **Child:** 10–20 mg/kg/d (max, 750–1,000 mg) PO in two equal div doses.
UTI—**Adult:** 250 mg PO q 12 h × 2 wk.

dapsone • Avlosulfon ◆

Synthetic sulfone; antileprotic, antimalarial
PRC: C

Tab: 25 mg, 100 mg

Multibacillary leprosy (with rifampin and clofazimine for 12 mo)—**Adult:** 100 mg/d PO. **Child 10–14 yr:** 50 mg/d PO. **Child < 10 yr:** 25 mg/d PO.
Paucibacillary leprosy (with rifampin for 6 mo)—**Adult:** 100 mg/d PO. **Child 10–14 yr:** 50 mg/d PO. **Child < 10 yr:** 25 mg/d PO.
Prophx for people in close contact with leprosy pt—**Adult, child ≥ 12 yr:** 50 mg/d PO. **Child 6–12 yr:** 25 mg/d PO. **Child 2–5 yr:** 25 mg PO 3 times/wk. **Infant 6–23 mo:** 12 mg PO 3 times/wk. **Infant < 6 mo:** 6 mg PO 3 times/wk.
Dermatitis herpetiformis—**Adult:** Initially, 50 mg/d PO;

(continued)

Classes	Dosage Forms	Indications & Dosages
dapsone *(continued)*		
		may incr to max of 300 mg/d PO for full control. *Malaria suppression or prophx*—**Adult:** 100 mg/wk PO with pyrimethamine 12.5 mg/wk PO. Cont prophx through and 6 mo after exposure. **Child:** 2 mg/kg/wk PO with pyrimethamine 0.25 mg/kg/wk. Cont prophx through and 6 mo after exposure. Pneumocystis carinii *pneumonia* ◇—**Adult:** 100 mg/d PO × 21 d, usually with trimethoprim 20 mg/kg/d. *Prophx of* P. carinii *pneumonia* ◇—**Adult:** 50 mg bid or 100 mg/d PO *Prophx of toxoplasmosis in HIV-infected pts* ◇—**Adult, adolescent:** 50 mg/d PO with pyrimethamine 50 mg and leucovorin 25 mg once/wk. **Child, infant ≥ 1 mo:** 2 mg/kg or 15 mg/m^2 (max, 25 mg) PO once/d plus pyrimethamine and leucovorin.
delavirdine mesylate • Rescriptor		
Non-nucleoside reverse-transcriptase inhibitor of HIV-1; antiviral PRC: C	*Tab:* 100 mg, 200 mg	*HIV infect*—**Adult:** 400 mg PO tid with other antiretrovirals.
dicloxacillin sodium • Dycill, Dynapen, Pathocil		
Penicillinase-resistant penicillin; antibiotic PRC: B	*Caps:* 125 mg, 250 mg, 500 mg; *Oral susp:* 62.5 mg/5 ml (after reconst)	*Systemic infect from penicillinase-producing staph*—**Adult, child weighing ≥ 40 kg:** 125–250 mg PO q 6 h. **Infant, child > 1 mo weighing < 40 kg:** 12.5–50 mg/kg/d PO, div and given q 6 h. Serious infect may warrant 75–100 mg/kg/d div doses q 6 h.

didanosine (ddI) • Videx, Videx EC

Purine analogue; antiviral PRC: B	*Caps (del-rel):* 125 mg, 200 mg, 250 mg, 400 mg; *Pwd oral sol (buffered):* 100, 167, 250 mg/packet; *Pwd oral sol (ped):* 2 g in 4-oz and 4 g in 8-oz bottles; *Tab (chew):* 25 mg, 50 mg, 100 mg, 150 mg, 200 mg	*HIV infect when antiretroviral therapy warranted*—**Adult ≥ 60 kg (132 lb):** 200 mg (tab) PO bid. Or, 400 mg (two 200-mg chew tab or one 400-mg del-rel caps) once/d. Or, 250 mg buffered powder PO bid. **Adult < 60 kg:** 125 mg (tab) PO bid Or, 250 mg (chew tab or del-rel caps) once/d. Or, 167 mg buffered powder PO bid. **Child:** 120 mg/m^2 PO bid. To prevent gastric acid degradation, give 2-tab dose to child > 1 and 1-tab dose to child < 1. Videx EC isn't for children. ≡ ***Dosage adjustment.*** Dosage may need adjustment for renal impairment.

dirithromycin • Dynabac

Macrolide; antibiotic PRC: C	*Tab (ent-coated):* 250 mg	*Acute bacterial exacer of chronic bronchitis from* Haemophilus influenzae, Moraxella catarrhalis, Streptococcus pneumoniae; *secondary bacterial infect of acute bronchitis from* M. catarrhalis, S. pneumoniae; *uncomplicated skin and skin structure infect from* S. pyogenes, Staphylococcus aureus *(methicillin susceptible)*—**Adult, child ≥ 12 yr:** 500 mg/d PO with food × 7 d. *Community-acquired pneumonia from* Legionella pneumophila, Mycoplasma pneumoniae, S. pneumoniae—**Adult, child ≥ 12 yr:** 500 mg/d PO with food × 14 d. *Pharyngitis or tonsillitis from* S. pyogenes—**Adult, child ≥ 12 yr:** 500 mg/d PO with food × 10 d.

docosanol • Abreva

Antiviral; antiviral PRC: D	*Cream:* 10%	*Recurrent oral-facial herpes simplex*—**Adult, child ≥ 12 yr:** Apply 5 times/d with first indication of episode and cont until lesion healed.

Classes	Dosage Forms	Indications & Dosages

doxycycline calcium • Vibramycin
doxycycline hyclate • Apo-Doxy ♦, Doryx, Doxy Caps, Doxy 100, Doxy 200, Doxychel Hyclate, Doxycin ♦, Novo-Doxylin ♦, Periostat, Vibramycin, Vibra-Tabs
doxycycline hydrochloride • Doryx, Doxylin, Vibramycin
doxycycline monohydrate • Monodox, Vibramycin

Classes	Dosage Forms	Indications & Dosages
Tetracycline; antibiotic PRC: D	**doxycycline calcium** *Oral susp:* 50 mg/5 ml; **doxycycline hyclate** *Caps:* 20 mg, 50 mg, 100 mg; Caps *(ent-coated pellets):* 100 mg; Inj: 100 mg, 200 mg; *Tab (film-coated):* 50 mg, 100 mg; **doxycycline hydrochloride** *Caps:* 50 mg‡, 100 mg‡; *Tab:* 50 mg‡, 100 mg‡; **doxycycline monohydrate** *Caps:* 50 mg, 100 mg; *Oral susp:* 25 mg/5 ml	*Infect from susceptible gram-pos, gram-neg organisms (including* Haemophilus ducreyi, Yersinia pestis, Campylobacter fetus*),* Rickettsiae sp., Mycoplasma pneumoniae, Chlamydia trachomatis, Borrelia burgdorferi *(Lyme disease); psittacosis; granuloma inguinale*—**Adult, child > 8 yr weighing ≥ 45 kg (99 lb):** 100 mg PO q 12 h on d 1; then 100 mg/d PO. Or, 200 mg IV on d 1 in 1–2 inf; then 100 to 200 mg/d IV. **Child > 8 yr weighing < 45 kg:** 4.4 mg/kg/d PO or IV in div doses q 12 h on d 1; then 2.2 to 4.4 mg/kg/d in one to two div doses. Give inf over ≥ 1 h and complete it ≤ 12 h (6 h in lactated Ringer's sol or dextrose 5% in lactated Ringer's sol). *Inhal, GI, oropharyngeal anthrax (with 1–2 other antibiotics)*—**Adult:** Initially, 100 mg IV q 12 h until susceptibility results known; then 100 mg PO bid × 60 d. **Child > 8 yr weighing > 45 kg:** Initially, 100 mg IV q 12 h; then 100 mg PO bid × 60 d. **Child > 8 yr weighing ≤ 45 kg:** Initially, 2.2 mg/kg IV q 12 h; then 2.2 mg/kg PO bid × 60 d. **Child ≤ 8 yr:** Initially, 2.2 mg/kg IV q 12 h; then 2.2 mg/kg PO bid. *Gonorrhea in pt allergic to PCN*—**Adult:** 100 mg PO bid × 7 d (10 d for epididymitis). *Primary or secondary syphilis in pts allergic to PCN*—**Adult:** 300 mg/d PO in div doses × ≥ 10 d. *Uncomplicated urethral, endocervical, or rectal infect from* C. trachomatis *or* Ureaplasma urealyticum—**Adult:** 100 mg PO bid × ≥ 7 d (10 d for epididymitis).

Prophx of malaria—**Adult:** 100 mg/d PO starting 1–2 days before travel to endemic area and cont 4 wk after travel. **Child > 8 yr:** 2 mg/kg PO once/d starting 1–2 d before travel to endemic area and cont 4 wk after travel. Max, 100 mg/d.
PID—**Adult:** 100 mg IV q 12 h with cefoxitin or cefotetan, cont ≥ 2 d after symptoms improve; then 100 mg PO q 12 h × 14 d.
Cutaneous anthrax—**Adult:** 100 mg PO bid × 60 d. **Child > 8 yr weighing > 45 kg:** 100 mg PO q 12 h × 60 d. **Child > 8 yr weighing ≤ 45 kg:** 2.2 mg/kg q 12 h PO × 60 d. **Child ≤ 8 yr:** 2.2 mg/kg q 12 h PO × 60 d.

drotrecogin alfa (activated) • Xigris

Recombinant human activated protein C; sepsis agent PRC: C	*Inj:* 5 mg, 20 mg	*Reduction of mortality in pts with severe sepsis (with acute organ dysfunction) at risk of death*—**Adult:** 24 mcg/kg/h IV inf × 96 h.

econazole nitrate • Spectazole

Synthetic imidazole derivative; antifungal PRC: C	*Cream:* 1% (water-soluble base)	*Cutaneous candidiasis*—**Adult, child:** Rub into affected areas in am and pm. *Tinea pedis, cruris, corporis, and versicolor*—**Adult, child:** Rub into affected area once/d.

efavirenz • Sustiva

Nonnucleoside, reverse transcriptase inhibitor; antiretroviral PRC: C	*Caps:* 50 mg, 100 mg, 200 mg	*HIV-1 infect (with protease inhibitor or nucleoside analogue reverse transcriptase inhibitors)*—**Adult:** 600 mg PO once/d. **Child ≥ 3 yr weighing ≥ 40 kg:** 600 mg PO once/d. **Child ≥ 3 yr weighing 33–39 kg:** 400 mg PO once/d. **Child ≥ 3 yr weighing 25–32 kg:** 350 mg PO once/d. **Child ≥ 3 yr weighing 20–24 kg:** 300 mg PO once/d. **Child ≥ 3 yr weighing 15–19 kg:** 250 mg PO once/d. **Child ≥ 3 yr weighing 10–14 kg:** 200 mg PO once/d.

Classes	Dosage Forms	Indications & Dosages
enoxacin • Penetrex		
Fluoroquinolone; antibiotic PRC: C	*Tab (film-coated):* 200 mg, 400 mg	*Uncomplicated UTI (cystitis) from* Escherichia coli, Staphylococcus epidermidis, Staphylococcus saprophyticus—**Adult:** 200 mg PO q 12 h × 7 d. *Complicated UTI from* E. coli, Klebsiella pneumoniae, Proteus mirabilis, Pseudomonas aeruginosa, S. epidermidis, Enterobacter cloacae—**Adult:** 400 mg PO q 12 h × 14 d. *Uncomplicated urethral or endocervical gonorrhea (*Neisseria gonorrhoeae*)*—**Adult:** 400 mg PO single dose. ≡ ***Dosage adjustment.*** If CrCl ≤ 30 ml/min, start with usual initial dose and reduce later doses by half.
ertapenem • INVANZ		
Carbapenem; antibiotic PRC: B	*Inj:* 1 g	*Complicated intra-abdominal infect*—**Adult:** 1 g IV or IM once/d × 5–14 d. *Complicated skin and skin-structure infect*—**Adult:** 1 g IV or IM once/d × 7–14 d. *Community-acquired pneumonia*—**Adult:** 1 g IV or IM once/d × 10–14 d. *Complicated UTI (including pyelonephritis)*—**Adult:** 1 g IV or IM once/d × 10–14 d. *Acute pelvic infect including postpartum endomyometritis, septic abortion, post-surgical gyn infect*—**Adult:** 1 g IV or IM once/d × 3–10 d ≡ ***Dosage adjustment.*** If CrCl ≤ 30 ml/min, give 500 mg/d. If given ≤ 6 h before hemodialysis, give suppl dose of 150 mg after session.

erythromycin base • Apo-Erythro base ◆, E-Base, E-Mycin, Erybid ◆, ERYC, Ery-Tab, Erythromid ◆, Erythromycin Base/Filmtabs, Ilotycin, Novo-Rythro ◆, PCE
erythromycin estolate • Ilosone, Novo-Rythro ◆
erythromycin ethylsuccinate • Apo-Erythro-ES ◆, E.E.S., E.E.S. Granules, EryPed, EryPed Drops, Pediazole
erythromycin gluceptate • Ilotycin
erythromycin lactobionate • Erythrocin
erythromycin stearate • Apo-Erythro-S ◆, Erythrocin Stearate Filmtab, Novo-Rythro ◆
erythromycin (topical) • Akne-Mycin, A/T/S, Del-Mycin, Erycette, EryDerm, Erygel, Erymax, Ery-Sol, Erythra-Derm, Staticin, Theramycin Z, T-Stat
erythromycin (ophth) • Ilotycin

Macrolide; antibiotic
PRC: B

erythromycin base *Caps (del-rel)*: 250 mg; *Tab (ent-coated)*: 250 mg, 333 mg, 500 mg; **erythromycin estolate** *Caps*: 250 mg; *Susp*: 125 mg/5 ml, 250 mg/5 ml; *Tab*: 500 mg; **erythromycin ethylsuccinate** *Granules oral susp*: 200 mg/5 ml (after reconst); *Oral susp*: 200 mg/5 ml, 400 mg/5 ml; *Pwd oral susp*: 100 mg/2.5 ml, 200 mg/5 ml, 400 mg/5 ml (after reconst); *Tab*: 400 mg; *Tab (chew)*: 200 mg;

Acute pelvic inflammatory disease from Neisseria gonorrhoeae—**Adult:** 500 mg IV (gluceptate, lactobionate) q 6 h × 3 d; then 250 mg (base, estolate, stearate) or 400 mg (ethylsuccinate) PO q 6 h × 7 d.

Intestinal amebiasis in pt who can't take metronidazole—**Adult:** 250 mg (base, estolate, stearate) or 400 mg (ethylsuccinate) PO q 6 h × 10–14 d. **Child:** 30–50 mg/kg/d (base, estolate, ethylsuccinate, stearate) PO, div q 6 h × 10–14 d.

Mild to moderately severe respiratory tract, skin, and soft-tissue infect—**Adult:** 250–500 mg (base, estolate, stearate) PO q 6 h. Or, 333 mg (base) PO q 8 h. Or, 400–800 mg (ethylsuccinate) PO q 6 h. Or, 15–20 mg/kg/d (gluceptate, lactobionate) IV in div doses q 6 h. **Child:** 30–50 mg/kg/d (erythromycin salts) PO in div doses q 6 h. Or, 15–20 mg/kg/d IV in div doses q 4–6 h.

Syphilis—**Adult:** 500 mg (base, estolate, stearate) PO qid × 14 d.

Legionnaire's disease—**Adult:** 500 mg–1 g IV or PO (base, estolate, stearate) or 800–1,600 mg (ethylsuccinate) PO q 6 h × 21 d.

Uncomplicated urethral, endocervical, or rectal infect when tetracyclines contraindicated—**Adult:** 500 mg (base, estolate, stearate) or 800 mg (ethylsuccinate) PO qid × ≥ 7 d.

(continued)

Classes	Dosage Forms	Indications & Dosages
erythromycin base **erythromycin estolate** **erythromycin ethylsuccinate** **erythromycin gluceptate** **erythromycin lactobionate** **erythromycin stearate** **erythromycin (topical)** **erythromycin (ophth)** *(continued)*		
	erythromycin gluceptate *Inj:* 500-mg, 1-g vials; **erythromycin lactobionate** *Inj:* 500-mg, 1-g vials **erythromycin stearate** *Tab (film-coated): 250* mg, 500 mg; **erythromycin (topical)** *Pledgets:* 2%; *Gel:* 2%; *Oint:* 2%; *Sol:* 1.5%, 2%; **erythromycin (ophth)** *Oint:* 0.5%	*Urogenital* Chlamydia trachomatis *infect during pregnancy*—**Adult:** 500 mg (base, estolate, stearate) PO qid × ≥ 7 days or 250 mg (base, estolate, stearate) or 400 mg (ethylsuccinate) PO qid × ≥ 14 d. *Conjunctivitis from* C. trachomatis—**Neonate:** 50 mg/kg/d PO in four div doses ≥ 2 wk. *Pneumonia in infancy from* C. trachomatis—**Infant:** 50 mg/kg/d PO in four div doses ≥ 3 wk. *Topical tx acne vulgaris*—**Adult, child:** Apply to affected area bid. *Prophx ophthalmia neonatorum*—**Neonate:** 1-cm ribbon of oint in lower conjunctival sac of each eye ≥ 1 h after birth. New tube for each infant. Don't flush after instillation. *Acute and chronic conjunctivitis, trachoma, other eye infect*—**Adult, child:** 1-cm ribbon of oint into infected eye up to 6 times/d based on severity.

ethambutol hydrochloride • Etibi ♦, Myambutol

Classes	Dosage Forms	Indications & Dosages
semisynthetic antituberculotic; antituberculotic PRC: NR	*Tab:* 100 mg, 400 mg	*Adjunct tx pulmonary TB*—**Adult, child ≥ 13 yr:** If no previous anti-TB therapy, 15 mg/kg/d PO as single dose initially. **Retreatment:** 25 mg/kg/d PO as single dose × 60 d with ≥ 1 other antituberculotics; then decrease to 15 mg/kg/d PO as single dose.

famciclovir • Famvir

Synthetic acyclic guanine derivative; antiviral
PRC: B

Tab: 125 mg, 250 mg, 500 mg

Mgt of acute herpes zoster, immunocompetent pt—**Adult:** 500 mg PO q 8 h × 7 d.
≡ ***Dosage adjustment.*** If CrCl 40–59 ml/min, give 500 mg q 12 h. If 20–39 ml/min, give 500 mg q 24 h. If < 20 ml/min, give 250 mg q 48 h.
Recurrent genital herpes, immunocompetent pt—**Adult:** 125 mg PO bid × 5 d.
Long-term suppressive therapy for recurrent genital herpes, immunocompetent pts—**Adult:** 250 mg PO q 12 h up to 1 yr.
≡ ***Dosage adjustment.*** If CrCl 40–59 ml/min, give 125 mg q 12 h. If 20–39 ml/min, give 125 mg q 24 h. If < 20 ml/min, give 125 mg q 48 h.
Long-term suppression or maint prophx of HSV infect in HIV-infect pt—**Adult:** 500 mg PO bid × 7 d.

fluconazole • DiFlucan

Bis-triazole derivative; antifungal
PRC: C

Inj: 200 mg/100 ml, 400 mg/200 ml; *Susp:* 10 mg/ml, 40 mg/ml; *Tab:* 50 mg, 100 mg, 150 mg, 200 mg

Oropharyngeal, esophageal candidiasis—**Adult:** 200 mg PO or IV day 1; then 100 mg PO or IV once/d. Up to 400 mg/d esophageal disease. Cont ≥ 2 wk after symptoms resolve. **Child:** 6 mg/kg day 1; then 3 mg/kg ≥ 2 wk.
Systemic candidiasis—**Adult:** Up to 400 mg PO or IV once/d. Cont ≥ 2 wk after symptoms resolve. **Child:** 6–12 mg/kg/d IV or PO.
Cryptococcal meningitis—**Adult:** 400 mg IV or PO day 1; then 200 mg once/d. Cont tx 10–12 wk after CSF culture negative. To suppress relapse in AIDS pt, give 200 mg once/d. **Child:** 12 mg/kg IV or PO day 1; then 6 mg/kg once/d × 10–12 wk.
Vaginal candidiasis—**Adult:** 150 mg PO single dose.
UTI, peritonitis—**Adult:** 50–200 mg/d PO or IV.
Prophx in pts having BMT—**Adult:** 400 mg/d PO or IV for several days before procedure and 7 days after neutrophil count > 1,000 cells/mm^3. *(continued)*

Classes	Dosage Forms	Indications & Dosages
fluconazole *(continued)*		
		Candidal infection, long-term suppression HIV-infect pt— **Adult:** 100–200 mg/d PO or IV. *Prophx for mucocutaneous candidiasis, cryptococcosis, coccidioidomycosis, histoplasmosis in HIV-infect pt* ◇ —**Adult:** 200–400 mg/d PO or IV. **Infant, child:** 2–8 mg/kg/d PO. ≡ ***Dosage adjustment***. Give ½ usual adult dose if CrCl 21–49 ml/min, ¼ if 11–20 ml/min. Give one full dose after hemodialysis.
flucytosine (5-FC) • Ancobon		
Fluorinated pyrimidine; antifungal PRC: C	*Caps:* 250 mg, 500 mg	*Severe fungal infect from susceptible strains of* Candida *and* Cryptococcus—**Adult:** 50–150 mg/kg/d PO in div doses q 6 h. *Chromomycosis* ◇ —**Adult:** 150 mg/kg/d PO. ≡ ***Dosage adjustment.*** Reduce dosage 20–80% if CrCl ≤ 50 ml/min. Or, incr to q 12 h if CrCl 20–40 ml/min, q 24 h if 10–20 ml/min, or q 24–48 h if < 10 ml/min. Monitor drug level. Hemodialysis and peritoneal dialysis remove drug; giving 20–50 mg/kg PO immed after hemodialysis q 2–3 d ensures therapeutic levels.
fomivirsen sodium • Vitravene		
Phosphorothioate oligonucleotide; antiviral PRC: C	*Intravitreal inj:* Preservative-free, single-use vials of 0.25 ml, 6.6 mg/ml	*Local tx of CMV retinitis in AIDS pt with intolerance, contraindication, or unresponsiveness to other tx*—**Adult:** Induction, 330 mcg (0.05 ml) by intravitreal inj every other wk for two doses. Then, for maint, 330 mcg (0.05 ml) by intravitreal inj once q 4 wk.
foscarnet sodium (phosphonoformic acid) • Foscavir		
Pyrophosphate ana-	*Inj:* 24 mg/ml in 250-ml	*CMV retinitis in AIDS pt*—**Adult:** Initially, 90 mg/kg IV inf over 1½–2 h q 12 h

logue; antiviral
PRC: C

and 500-ml vials

or 60 mg/kg IV inf over 1 h q 8 h × 2–3 wk as induction tx in pt with normal renal function. Follow with maint inf of 90–120 mg/kg/d given over 2 h; incr as needed and tolerated to 120 mg/kg/d if disease progresses. Dosage based on renal function.

Mucocutaneous acyclovir-resistant HSV infect—**Adult:** 40 mg/kg IV inf over 1 h q 8–12 h × 2–3 wk, depending on response.

≡ ***Dosage adjustment.*** For adults with renal impairment, calculate weight-adjusted CrCl (ml/min/kg). For men, CrCl = (140 – age) / (serum creatinine × 72). For women, multiply above value by 0.85.

Mgt of HSV infect (equiv to 80 mg/kg/d [40 mg/kg q 12 h]): Give 40 mg q 12 h if CrCl > 1.4 ml/min/kg, 30 mg q 12 h if > 1–1.4 ml/min/kg, 20 mg q 12 h if > 0.8–1 ml/min/kg, 35 mg q 24 h if > 0.6–0.8 ml/min/kg, 25 mg q 24 h if > 0.5–0.6 ml/min/kg, and 20 mg q 24 h if 0.4–0.5 ml/min/kg. Avoid if CrCl is < 0.4 ml/min/kg.

Mgt of HSV infect (equiv to 120 mg/kg/d [40 mg/kg q 8 h]): Give 40 mg q 8 h if CrCl > 1.4 ml/min/kg, 30 mg q 8 h if > 1–1.4 ml/min/kg, 35 mg q 12 h if > 0.8–1 ml/min/kg, 25 mg q 12 h if > 0.6–0.8 ml/min/kg, 40 mg q 24 h if > 0.5–0.6 ml/min/kg, 35 mg q 24 h if 0.4–0.5 ml/min/kg. Avoid if CrCl is < 0.4 ml/min/kg.

Mgt of CMV (induction, equiv 180 mg/kg/d [60 mg/kg q 8 h]): Give 60 mg q 8 h if CrCl > 1.4 ml/min/kg, 45 mg q 8 h if > 1–1.4 ml/min/kg, 50 mg q 12 h if > 0.8–1 ml/min/kg, 40 mg q 12 h if > 0.6–0.8 ml/min/kg, 60 mg q 24 h if > 0.5–0.6 ml/min/kg, 50 mg q 24 h if 0.4–0.5 ml/min/kg. Avoid if CrCl < 0.4 ml/min/kg.

Mgt of CMV (induction, equiv 180 mg/kg/d [90 mg/kg q 12 h]): Give 90 mg q 12 h if CrCl > 1.4 ml/min/kg, 70 mg q 12 h if > 1–1.4 ml/min/kg, 50 mg q 12 h if > 0.8–1 ml/min/kg, 80 mg q 24 h if > 0.6–0.8 ml/min/kg, 60 mg q 24 h if > 0.5–0.6 ml/min/kg, 50 mg q 24 h if 0.4–0.5 ml/min/kg. Avoid if < 0.4 ml/min/kg.

(continued)

Classes	Dosage Forms	Indications & Dosages
foscarnet sodium (phosphonoformic acid) *(continued)*		
		Mgt of CMV (maint, equiv 90 mg/kg/d [once/d]): Give 90 mg q 24 h if CrCl > 1.4 ml/min/kg, 70 mg q 24 h if > 1–1.4 ml/kg/min, 50 mg q 24 h if > 0.8–1 ml/min/kg, 80 mg q 48 h if > 0.6–0.8 ml/min/kg, 60 mg q 48 h if > 0.5–0.6 ml/min/kg, 50 mg q 48 h if 0.4–0.5 ml/min/kg. Avoid if CrCl < 0.4 ml/min/kg. *Mgt of CMV (maint, equiv 120 mg/kg/d [once/d]):* Give 120 mg q 24 h if CrCl > 1.4 ml/min/kg, 90 mg q 24 h if > 1–1.4 ml/min/kg, 65 mg q 24 h if > 0.8–1 ml/min/kg, 105 mg q 48 h if > 0.6–0.8 ml/min/kg, 80 mg q 48 h if > 0.5–0.6 ml/min/kg, 65 mg q 48 h if 0.4–0.5 ml/min/kg. Avoid if CrCl < 0.4 ml/min/kg.
ganciclovir (DHPG) • Cytovene		
Synthetic nucleoside; antiviral PRC: C	*Caps:* 250 mg, 500 mg; *Inj:* 500-mg vial	*CMV retinitis*—**Adult:** Initially, 5 mg/kg IV q 12 h × 14–21 d; then maint of 5 mg/kg IV once/d × 7 d/wk or 6 mg/kg IV once/d × 5 d/wk. Give inf at constant rate over 1 h. Or, maint of 1,000 mg PO tid or 500 mg PO q 3 h while awake (6 times/d). *Prophx of CMV after transplant*—**Adult:** 5 mg/kg IV over 1 h q 12 h × 7–14 d; then maint of 5 mg/kg once/d × 7 d/wk or 6 mg/kg once/d × 5 d/wk. *Other CMV infect*◇—**Adult:** 5 mg/kg IV over 1 h q 12 h × 14–21 d. Or, 2.5 mg/kg IV q 8 h × 14–21 d. ≡ ***Dosage adjustment.*** Give 2.5 mg/kg q 12 h if CrCl is 50–69 ml/min, 2.5 mg/kg q 24 h if 25–49 ml/min, 1.25 mg/kg q 24 h if 10–24 ml/min, or 1.25 mg/kg 3 times/wk if < 10 ml/min or just after hemodialysis.
gatifloxacin • Tequin		
Fluoroquinolone; antibiotic PRC: C	*Inj:* 200 mg/20-ml vial, 400 mg/40-ml vial, 200 mg in 100 ml D_5W,	*Complicated UTI from* Escherichia coli, Klebsiella pneumoniae, *or* Proteus mirabilis; *acute pyelonephritis from* E. coli—**Adult:** 400 mg/d IV or PO × 7–10 d.

	400 mg in 200 ml D_5W; *Tab:* 200 mg, 400 mg	*Acute bacterial exacer of chronic bronchitis from* Streptococcus pneumoniae, Haemophilus influenzae, H. parainfluenzae, Moraxella catarrhalis, *or* Staphylococcus aureus—**Adult:** 400 mg/d IV or PO × 5 d. *Acute sinusitis from* S. pneumoniae *or* H. influenzae—**Adult:** 400 mg/d IV or PO × 10 d. *Community-acquired pneumonia from* S. pneumoniae, H. influenzae, H. parainfluenzae, M. catarrhalis, S. aureus, Mycoplasma pneumoniae, Chlamydia pneumoniae, *or* Legionella pneumophila—**Adult:** 400 mg/d IV or PO × 7–14 d. *Uncomplicated urethral gonorrhea (men), cervical gonorrhea or acute uncomplicated rectal infect (women) from* Neisseria gonorrhoeae—**Adult:** 400 mg PO or IV as single dose. *Uncomplicated UTI from* E. coli, K. pneumoniae, *or* P. mirabilis—**Adult:** 400 mg IV or PO as single dose, or 200 mg/d IV or PO × 3 d. ≡ ***Dosage adjustment.*** Initially, 400 mg/d and then 200 mg/d IV or PO if CrCl < 40 ml/min or pt receives hemodialysis or cont peritoneal dialysis. If pt receives hemodialysis, give drug after session complete.

gentamicin sulfate • Cidomycin ◆, G-myticin, Garamycin, Genoptic, Genoptic S.O.P., Gentacidin, Gentafair, Gentak, Gentasol, Jenamicin

Aminoglycoside; antibiotic PRC: D	*Inj:* 40 mg/ml (adult), 10 mg/ml (ped), 2 mg/ml (intrathecal); *Ophth oint:* 3 mg/g; *Ophth sol:* 3 mg/ml; *Topical cream, oint:* 0.1%	*Serious infect*—**Adult:** 3 mg/kg/d IM or IV inf over ½–2 h (in 50–100 ml NSS or D_5W) div doses q 8 h. Up to 5 mg/kg/d in three to four div doses if life-threatening. **Child:** 2 to 2.5 mg/kg IM or IV inf q 8 h. **Infant, neonate > 1 wk:** 2.5 mg/kg IM or IV inf q 8 h. **Neonate ≤ 1 wk:** 2.5 mg/kg IM or IV inf q 12 h. For inf, dilute in NSS or D_5W and inf over ½–2 h. *Meningitis*—**Adult:** As above; or 4–8 mg/d intrathecal. **Child:** As above; or 1–2 mg/d intrathecal. *Prophx of endocarditis for GI or GU procedure or surg (with ampicillin)*—**Adult:** 1.5 mg/kg IM or IV 30 min before procedure and 6 h after. **Child:** 2 mg/kg IM or IV 30 min before procedure and 6 h after.

(continued)

Classes	Dosage Forms	Indications & Dosages
gentamicin sulfate *(continued)*		
		External ocular infect—**Adult, child:** 1–2 gtt in eye q 4 h. Up to 2 gtt q h for serious infect. Oint in lower conjunctival sac bid or tid. *Primary, secondary bacterial infect; superficial burn; skin ulcer; infected laceration, abrasion, insect bite, minor surg wound*—**Adult, child > 1:** Small amt tid or qid, maybe with gauze dressing. *Pelvic inflammatory disease*—**Adult:** Initially, 2 mg/kg IM or IV. Then 1.5 mg/kg q 8 h. ≡ ***Dosage adjustment.*** Initial dose unchanged. Later doses based on renal function and blood level. Keep peak serum level at 4–10 mcg/ml and trough at 1–2 mcg/ml. After hemodialysis to keep therapeutic levels—**Adult:** 1–1.7 mg/kg IM or IV inf. **Child:** 2–2.5 mg/kg IM or IV inf.
griseofulvin microsize • Fulvicin U/F, Grifulvin V, Grisactin **griseofulvin ultramicrosize** • Fulvicin P/G, Grisactin Ultra, Gris-PEG		
Penicillium antibiotic; antifungal PRC: C	**microsize** *Caps:* 250 mg; *Oral susp:* 125 mg/5 ml; *Tab:* 250 mg, 500 mg; **ultramicrosize** *Tab:* 125 mg, 165 mg, 250 mg, 330 mg; *Tab (film-coated):* 125 mg, 250 mg	*Tinea corporis, capitis, barbae, or cruris*—**Adult:** 330 mg/d PO ultramicrosize or 500 mg/d PO microsize. **Child weighing 14–23 kg (30–50 lb):** 82.5–165 mg/d PO ultramicrosize or 125–250 mg/d PO microsize. **Child weighing > 23 kg:** 165–330 mg/d PO ultramicrosize or 250–500 mg/d PO microsize. *Tinea pedis or unguium*—**Adult:** 660 mg/d PO ultramicrosize or 1 g/d PO microsize. **Child weighing 14–23 kg (30–50 lb):** 82.5–165 mg/d PO ultramicrosize or 125–250 mg/d PO microsize. **Child weighing > 23 kg:** 165–330 mg/d PO ultramicrosize or 250–500 mg/d PO microsize.
hydroxychloroquine sulfate • Plaquenil		
4-aminoquinoline; antimalarial, anti-	*Tab:* 200 mg (155 mg base)	*Suppressive prophx of malarial attack*—**Adult:** 400 mg/wk sulfate (310 mg base) PO on same day each wk. Start 2 wk before entering area and cont 8 wk

inflammatory PRC: C		after leaving. **Infant, child:** 5 mg, calculate as base/kg body weight (max, adult dose) on same day each wk. Start 2 weeks before exposure. If unable, give 10 mg base/kg in two div doses 6 h apart. *Acute malaria attack*—**Adult:** 800 mg (620 mg base); then 400 mg (310 mg base) in 6–8 h and 400 mg (310 mg base) on each of 2 consecutive days. **Infant, child:** First dose, 10 mg base/kg (max, 620 mg base). Second dose, 5 mg base/kg (max, 310 mg base) 6 h after first dose. Third dose, 5 mg base/kg 18 h after second dose. Fourth dose, 5 mg base/kg 24 h after third dose. *Lupus erythematosus (chronic discoid, systemic)*—**Adult:** 400 mg PO once/d or bid, cont several wk or mo based on response. For prolonged maint, 200–400 mg/d PO. *Rheumatoid arthritis*—**Adult:** 400–600 mg/d PO; after good response (usually 4–12 wk), cut dose in half.

imipenem and cilastatin sodium • Primaxin I.M., Primaxin I.V.

Carbapenem (thienamycin class), beta-lactam antibiotic; antibiotic PRC: C	*Inj:* 250-mg vial, 500-mg vial, ADD-Vantage, inf bottle; *Pwd for IM inj:* 500-mg vial, 750-mg vial	*Mild-to-moderate lower respiratory tract, skin and skin-structure, or gyn infect*—**Adult weighing ≥ 70 kg (154 lb):** 500–750 mg IM q 12 h. *Mild-to-moderate intra-abdominal infect*—**Adult weighing ≥ 70 kg:** 750 mg IM q 12 h. *Serious respiratory and urinary tract infect; intra-abdominal, gyn, bone, joint, or skin infect; bacterial septicemia; endocarditis*—**Adult weighing ≥ 70 kg:** 250 mg to 1 g IV inf q 6–8 h. Max, the smaller of 50 mg/kg/d or 4 g/d. **Child:** 15–25 mg/kg q 6 h. ≡ ***Dosage adjustment.*** 125–250 mg IV q 12 h for most pathogens if CrCl 6–20 ml/min (risk of seizures may incr at 500 mg q 12 h). Avoid drug if CrCl ≤ 5 ml/min unless hemodialysis given within 48 h. Dosage varies if pt weighs < 70 kg.

Classes	Dosage Forms	Indications & Dosages
indinavir sulfate • Crixivan		
HIV protease inhibitor; antiviral PRC: C	*Caps:* 100 mg, 200 mg, 333 mg, 400 mg	*HIV-infect when antiretroviral warranted*—**Adult:** 800 mg PO q 8 h with other antiretrovirals. Not used alone.
isoniazid (INH) • Isotamine ♦, Laniazid, Nydrazid, PMS Isoniazid ♦		
Isonicotinic acid hydrazine; antituberculotic PRC: C	*Inj:* 100 mg/ml; *Oral sol:* 50 mg/5 ml; *Tab:* 50 mg, 100 mg, 300 mg	*Primary tx against actively growing tubercle bacilli*—**Adult:** 5 mg/kg/d single dose PO or IM, up to 300 mg/d, × 9 mo to 2 yr. **Infant, child:** 10 mg/kg/d single dose PO or IM, up to 300 mg/d, × 18 mo to 2 yr. Use of at least one other antituberculotic recommended. *Prophx against tubercle bacilli in those closely exposed or with positive skin test*—**Adult:** 300 mg/d single dose PO for 6 mo to 1 yr. **Infant, child:** 10 mg/kg/d single dose PO, up to 300 mg daily, for 6 mo to 1 yr.
itraconazole • Sporanox		
Synthetic triazole; antifungal PRC: C	*Caps:* 100 mg; *Inj:* 10 mg/ml; *Oral sol:* 10 mg/ml	*Blastomycosis (pulmonary, extrapulmonary), histoplasmosis (including chronic cavitary pulmonary disease, disseminated nonmeningeal histoplasmosis)*—**Adult:** 200 mg PO once/d. If condition doesn't improve, incr dose in 100-mg steps to max of 400 mg/d. Give amt above 200 mg/d in two div doses. Or, 200 mg IV bid for four doses; then decr to 200 mg IV once/d for up to 14 d. *Aspergillosis (pulmonary, extrapulmonary) in pts intolerant of or refractory to amphotericin B*—**Adult:** 200–400 mg/d PO or 200 mg IV bid for four doses; then decr to 200 mg/d IV for up to 14 d. *Oropharyngeal candidiasis*—**Adult:** 200 mg/d (20 ml) oral sol PO × 1–2 wk. *Esophageal candidiasis*—**Adult:** 100 mg/d (10 ml) oral sol PO × ≥ 3 wk. *Superficial mycoses (dermatophytoses, pityriasis versicolor, sebopsoriasis,*

candidiasis [vaginal, oral, chronic mucocutaneous], onychomycosis) ◇, *leishmaniasis* ◇, *fungal keratitis* ◇, *alternariatoxicosis* ◇, *zygomycosis* ◇, *systemic mycoses (candidiasis, cryptococcal infect [meningitis, disseminated], dimorphic infect [paracoccidioidomycosis, coccidioidomycosis])* ◇, *SC mycoses (sporotrichosis, cutaneous chromomycosis)* ◇—**Adult:** 50–400 mg/d PO × 1 d to > 6 mo depending on condition and response.

ketoconazole • Nizoral

Imidazole derivative; antifungal
PRC: C

Cream: 2%; *Shampoo:* 2%; *Tab:* 200 mg

Severe fungal infect—**Adult:** Initially, 200 mg/d PO single dose. May incr to 400 mg once/d if no response to lower amt. **Child > 2 yr:** 3.3–6.6 mg/kg/d PO single dose.
Topical tx of tinea corporis, cruris, versicolor, pedis—**Adult, child:** Apply daily or bid × about 2 wk; for tinea pedis, 6 wk.
Seborrheic dermatitis—**Adult, child:** Apply bid × about 4 wk.
Dandruff—**Adult:** Apply for 1 min, rinse, then reapply for 3 min. Shampoo twice/wk × 4 wk, with ≥ 3 days between shampoos.
Prostatic carcinoma ◇, *disseminated intravascular coagulation related to prostatic cancer* ◇—**Adult:** 400 mg PO q 8 h.

lamivudine (3TC) • Epivir, Epivir-HBV

Synthetic nucleoside analogue; antiviral
PRC: C

Epivir *Oral sol:* 10 mg/ml; Tab: 150 mg; **Epivir-HBV** *Oral sol:* 5 mg/ml; Tab: 100 mg

HIV infect (tx with other antiretrovirals)—**Adult weighing ≥ 50 kg, adolescent ≥ 16 yr:** 150 mg PO bid. **Adult weighing < 50 kg:** 2 mg/kg PO bid. **Child, infant ≥ 3 mo:** 4 mg/kg PO bid. Max, 150 mg bid. **Neonate ≤ 1 mo** ◇: 2 mg/kg PO bid.

≡ ***Dosage adjustment.*** For adults and adolescents give 150 mg once/d if CrCl 30–49 ml/min; 150 mg first dose, then 100 mg once/d if 15–29 ml/min; 150 mg first dose, then 50 mg once/d if 5–14 ml/min; 50 mg first dose, then 25 mg once/d if < 5 ml/min. In children, consider decr dose or incr interval.

(continued)

Classes	Dosage Forms	Indications & Dosages
lamivudine (3TC) *(continued)*		
		Chronic hepatitis B with evidence of hepatitis B viral replication and active liver inflammation—**Adult:** 100 mg PO once/d. **Child 2–17 yr:** 3 mg/kg once/d to a max dose of 100 mg. ≡ ***Dosage adjustment.*** In pt ≥ 16, give 100 mg PO on day 1, then 50 mg PO once/d if CrCl 30–49 ml/min; 100 mg on day 1, then 25 mg PO once/d if 15–29 ml/min; 35 mg on day 1, then 15 mg once/d if 5–14 ml/min; 35 mg on day 1, then 10 mg PO once/d if < 5 ml/min. *Prophx after work exposure to HIV*◊—**Adult:** 150 mg PO bid with oral zidovudine (600 mg/d); indinavir (800 mg PO q 8 h) or nelfinavir (750 mg PO tid) added if high risk of transmission. Start within a few h and cont 28 d.
lamivudine and zidovudine • Combivir		
Reverse transcriptase inhibitor; antiretroviral PRC: C	*Tab:* 150 mg lamivudine and 300 mg zidovudine	*HIV infect*—**Adult, child > 12 yr weighing ≥ 50 kg:** One tab PO bid.
levofloxacin • Levaquin, Quixin		
Fluorinated carboxyquinolone; broad-spectrum antibiotic PRC: C	*Inf (premixed):* 250 mg in 50 ml D_5W, 500 mg in 100 ml D_5W, 750 mg in 150 ml D_5W; *Ophth sol:* 0.5%; *Single-use vial:* 500 mg, 750 mg; *Tab:* 250 mg, 500 mg, 750 mg	*Acute maxillary sinusitis from* Streptococcus pneumoniae, Moraxella catarrhalis, *or* Haemophilus influenzae—**Adult:** 500 mg/d PO or IV × 10–14 d. *Acute bacterial exacer of chronic bronchitis from* Staphylococcus aureus, S. pneumoniae, M. catarrhalis, H. influenzae, *or* Haemophilus parainfluenzae—**Adult:** 500 mg/d PO or IV × 7 d. *Community-acquired pneumonia from* S. aureus, S. pneumoniae, M. catarrhalis, H. influenzae, H. parainfluenzae, Klebsiella pneumoniae, Chlamydia pneumoniae, Legionella pneumoniae, *or* Mycoplasma pneumoniae—**Adult:** 500 mg/d PO or IV × 7–14 d.

Mild-to-moderate uncomplicated skin, skin-structure infect from S. aureus *or* Streptococcus pyogenes—**Adult:** 500 mg/d PO or IV × 7–10 d.

≡ ***Dosage adjustment.*** Initial dose 500 mg, later doses 250 mg if CrCl 20–49 ml/min. Later doses half of initial dose q 48 h if CrCl 10–19 ml/min.

Mild-to-moderate complicated UTI from Enterococcus faecalis, Enterobacter cloacae, Escherichia coli, K. pneumoniae, Proteus mirabilis, *or* Pseudomonas aeruginosa—**Adult:** 250 mg/d PO or IV × 10 d.

Mild-to-moderate acute pyelonephritis from E. coli—**Adult:** 250 mg/d PO or IV × 10 d.

≡ ***Dosage adjustment.*** Incr interval to q 48 h if CrCl 10–19 ml/min.

Traveler's diarrhea ◇—**Adult:** 500 mg PO single dose with loperamide hydrochloride.

Prophx of traveler's diarrhea ◇—**Adult:** 500 mg PO once/d during period of risk for up to 3 wk.

Complicated skin, skin-structure infect from methicillin-sensitive S. aureus, E. faecalis, S. pyogenes, or P. mirabilis—**Adult:** 750 mg PO once/d × 7–14 d.

Bacterial conjuctivitis from S. aureus, Staphylococcus epidermidis, S. pneumoniae, Streptococcus *(Groups C, F, G, Viridans),* Acinetobacter iwoffii, H. influenzae, *or* Serratia marcescens—**Adult:** For days 1–2, 1–2 gtt to affected eye q 2 h up to 8 times/d while awake. For days 3–7, 1–2 gtt to affected eye q 4 h up to 4 times/d while awake.

Community-acquired pneumonia from penicillin-resistant S. pneumoniae—**Adult:** 500 mg PO or IV inf over 60 min once/d × 7–14 d.

≡ ***Dosage adjustment.*** Initial dose of 500 mg, then 250 mg once/d if CrCl 20–49 ml/min. Initial dose of 500 mg, then 250 mg q 48 h if CrCl 10–19 ml/min. Initial dose of 500 mg, then 250 mg every 48 h if pt receiving hemodialysis or long-term ambulatory peritoneal dialysis.

Complicated skin, skin-structure infect from methicillin-sensitive S. aureus, E. faecalis, S. pyogenes, P. mirabilis—**Adult:** 750 mg PO *(continued)*

Classes	Dosage Forms	Indications & Dosages
levofloxacin *(continued)*		
		or IV inf over 90 min q 24 h × 7–14 d. ≡ ***Dosage adjustment.*** Give 750 mg initially, then 750 mg q 48 h if CrCl 20–49 ml/min. Give 750 mg initially, then 500 mg q 48 h if CrCl 10–19 ml/min or pt is receiving hemodialysis or long-term ambulatory peritoneal dialysis.
linezolid • Zyvox		
Oxazolidinone; antibiotic PRC: C	*Inj:* 2 mg/ml; *Pwd for oral susp:* 100 mg/5 ml when constituted; *Tab:* 400 mg, 600 mg	*Vancomycin-resistant* Enterococcus faecium *infect, including those with concurrent bacteremia*—**Adult:** 600 mg IV or PO q 12 h 3 14–28 d. *Nosocomial pneumonia from* Staphylococcus aureus *(methicillin-susceptible [MSSA] and methicillin-resistant [MRSA] strains) or* Streptococcus pneumoniae *(penicillin-susceptible strains only); complicated skin, skin-structure infect from* S. aureus *(MSSA and MRSA),* Streptococcus pyogenes, *or* Streptococcus agalactiae; *community-acquired pneumonia from* S. pneumoniae *(penicillin-susceptible strains only), including those with concurrent bacteremia, or* S. aureus *(MSSA only)*—**Adult:** 600 mg IV or PO q 12 h × 10–14 d. *Uncomplicated skin, skin-structure infect from* S. aureus *(MSSA only) or* S. pyogenes—**Adult:** 400 mg PO q 12 h × 10–14 d.
lopinavir and ritonavir • Kaletra		
Protease inhibitor; antiviral PRC: C	*Caps:* lopinavir 133.3 mg and ritonavir 33.3 mg; *Sol:* lopinavir 400 mg and ritonavir 100 mg/ 5 ml (80 mg/20 mg per ml)	*HIV infect (combined with other antiretrovirals)*—**Adult, child > 12 yr:** 400 mg lopinavir and 100 mg ritonavir (3 caps or 5 ml) PO bid with food. If probable reduced susceptibility to lopinavir (tx-experienced pt also taking efavirenz or nevirapine) may give 533/133 mg (4 caps or 6.5 ml) PO bid with food. **Child 6 mo–12 yr weighing 15–40 kg:** 10 mg/kg (lopinavir) PO bid with food. Max 400/100 mg in child weighing > 40 kg. If probable reduced susceptibility to lopinavir (tx-experienced pt also taking efavirenz or nevirapine weighing

15–50 kg) may give 11 mg/kg (lopinavir) PO bid (adult dose if child weighs > 50 kg). **Child 6 mo–12 yr weighing 7–14 kg:** 12 mg/kg (lopinavir) PO bid with food. If probable reduced susceptibility to lopinavir (tx-experienced pt also taking efavirenz or nevirapine) may give 13 mg/kg (lopinavir) PO bid with food.

loracarbef • Lorabid

Synthetic beta-lactam antibiotic of carba-cephem class; antibiotic PRC: B	*Pwd for oral susp:* 100 mg/5 ml, 200 mg/5 ml; *Pulvules:* 200 mg, 400 mg	*Secondary bacterial infect of acute bronchitis*—**Adult, adolescent ≥ 13 yr:** 200–400 mg PO q 12 h × 7 d. *Acute bacterial exacer of chronic bronchitis*—**Adult, adolescent ≥ 13 yr:** 400 mg PO q 12 h × 7 d. *Pneumonia*—**Adult, adolescent ≥ 13 yr:** 400 mg PO q 12 h × 14 d. *Pharyngitis, tonsillitis*—**Adult, adolescent ≥ 13 yr:** 200 mg PO q 12 h × 10 d. Child 6 mo to 12 yr: 15 mg/kg/d PO div doses q 12 h × 10 d. *Sinusitis*—**Adult, adolescent ≥ 13 yr:** 400 mg PO q 12 h × 10 d. Child 6 mo to 12 yr: 15 mg/kg PO q 12 h × 10 d. *Acute otitis media*—**Child 6 mo–12 yr:** 30 mg/kg/d (oral susp) div doses q 12 h × 10 d. *Uncomplicated skin, skin-structure infect*—**Adult, adolescent ≥ 13 yr:** 200 mg PO q 12 h × 7 d. *Impetigo*—**Child:** 15 mg/kg/d PO div doses q 12 h × 7 d. *Uncomplicated cystitis*—**Adult, adolescent ≥ 13 yr:** 200 mg/d PO × 7 d. *Uncomplicated pyelonephritis*—**Adult, adolescent ≥ 13 yr:** 400 mg PO q 12 h × 14 d. ≡ ***Dosage adjustment.*** If CrCl 10–49 ml/min, give half usual dose at usual interval or give usual dose at twice usual interval. If CrCl < 10 ml/min, give usual dose q 3–5 d. Give another dose after hemodialysis.

Classes	Dosage Forms	Indications & Dosages
mefloquine hydrochloride • Lariam		
Quinine derivative; antimalarial PRC: C	*Tab:* 250 mg	*Acute malaria infect from mefloquine-sensitive* Plasmodium falciparum, P. vivax—**Adult, child:** 15 mg/kg PO single dose; then second dose 10 mg/kg PO 6–8 h later. Max total dose, 1,250 mg. Pt with *P. vivax* infect should receive primaquine or other 8-aminoquinoline to avoid relapse after tx of initial infect. *Malaria prophx*—**Adult, child > 45 kg:** 250 mg PO once/wk. Prophx starts 1 wk before entering endemic area and cont 4 wk after returning. If pt returns without malaria after long stay in endemic area, prophx should end after three doses. **Child 31–45 kg:** 187.5 mg PO once/wk. **Child 20–30 kg:** 125 mg PO once/wk. **Child 15–19 kg:** 62.5 mg PO once/wk. **Child < 15 kg:** 5 mg/kg PO once/wk.
meropenem • Merrem IV		
Carbapenem derivative; antibiotic PRC: B	*Pwd for inj:* 500 mg/15 ml, 500 mg/20 ml, 500 mg/100 ml, 1 g/15 ml, 1 g/30 ml, 1 g/100 ml	*Complicated appendicitis and peritonitis from viridans group* streptococci, Escherichia coli, Klebsiella pneumoniae, Pseudomonas aeruginosa, Bacteroides fragilis, B. thetaiotaomicron, Peptostreptococcus *sp.; bacterial meningitis caused by* Streptococcus pneumoniae, Haemophilus influenzae, Neisseria meningitidis—Avoid conc above 50 mg/ml. **Adult:** 1 g IV q 8 h over 15–30 min as inf or over about 3–5 min as bolus inj (5–20 ml). **Child ≥ 3 mo and weighing ≤ 50 kg:** 20 mg/kg (intra-abdominal infect) or 40 mg/kg (bacterial meningitis) q 8 h over 15–30 min as inf or over about 3–5 min as bolus inj (5–20 ml). **Child weighing > 50 kg:** 1 g q 8 h for intra-abdominal infect; 2 g q 8 h for meningitis. ≡ ***Dosage adjustment.*** 1 g q 12 h if CrCl 26–50 ml/min, 500 mg q 12 h if 10–25 ml/min, and 500 mg q 24 h if < 10 ml/min. No experience with children.

metronidazole • Apo-Metronidazole ♦, Flagyl, Flagyl ER, Metric 21, Novonidazol ♦, Protostat
metronidazole hydrochloride • Flagyl IV, Flagyl IV RTU, Metro I.V.

Nitroimidazole; antibiotic, antiprotozoal, amebicide
PRC: B

Caps: 375 mg; *Inj:* 500 mg/dl ready to use; *Pwd for inj:* 500-mg single-dose vials; *Tab:* 250 mg, 500 mg; *Tab (ext-rel, film-coated):* 750 mg; *Tab (film-coated):* 250 mg, 500 mg

Amoebic hepatic abscess—**Adult:** 500–750 mg PO tid × 5–10 d. Or, 2.4 g/d PO × 1–2 d or 500 mg IV q 6 h × 10 d. **Child:** 30–50 mg/kg/d PO in three div doses × 5–10 d. Or, 1.3 $g/m^2/d$ PO in three div doses × 5–10 d.

Intestinal amebiasis—**Adult:** 750 mg PO tid × 5–10 d. CDC also recommends iodoquinol 650 mg PO tid × 20 d. Or, 2.4 g/d PO × 1–2 d or 500 mg IV q 6 h × 10 d. **Child** ◇**:** 30–50 mg/kg/d PO in three div doses × 5–10 d. Follow with oral iodoquinol. Or, 1.3 $g/m^2/d$ PO in three div doses × 5–10 d.

Trichomoniasis—**Adult (sexual partners concurrently):** 375-mg caps PO bid × 7 d, or 500-mg tab PO bid × 7 d, or single dose of 2 g PO or div into two doses on same day. **Child** ◇**:** 15 mg/kg/d PO in three div doses × 7–10 d. Or, 40 mg/kg PO single dose. Max dose, 2 g. **Infant > 4 wk** ◇**:** 10–30 mg/kg/d PO × 5–8 d.

Refractory trichomoniasis—**Woman:** 500 mg PO bid × 7 d. If repeated failure, 2 g/d PO × 3–5 d. Or (for repeated failure), 2–3.5 g/d PO × 3–21 d based on in vitro susceptibility test.

Bacterial infect from anaerobic organism—**Adult:** Loading dose, 15 mg/kg IV inf over 1 h (about 1 g for 70-kg adult). Maint, 7.5 mg/kg IV or PO q 6 h (about 500 mg for 70-kg adult). Give first maint dose 6 h after loading dose. Max, 4 g/d. Cont tx 7 d to 3 wk.

Giardiasis ◇ —**Adult:** 250 mg PO tid × 5 d, or 2 g once/d × 3 d. If coexistent amebiasis, 750 mg PO tid × 5–10 d. **Child:** 5 mg/kg PO tid × 5–7 d.

Prev of postop infect in contaminated or potentially contaminated colorectal surg—**Adult:** 15 mg/kg inf over 30–60 min and completed about 1 h before surg. Then 7.5 mg/kg inf over 30–60 min at 6 and 12 h after initial dose. If used with oral neomycin or oral kanamycin, 750 mg.

(continued)

Classes	Dosage Forms	Indications & Dosages
metronidazole **metronidazole hydrochloride** *(continued)*		
		PO bid to tid starting 2 d before surg. Or, 500 mg to 1 g IV 1 h before surg; then 500 mg IV at 8 and 16 h after surg. *Bacterial vaginosis*◇—**Adult:** 500 mg PO bid × 7 d. Or, 2 g PO single dose. Or, 750 mg/d (ext-rel) PO × 7 d. During pregnancy, 250 mg PO tid × 7 d or 2 g PO single dose. *PID*—**Adult:** 500 mg IV q 12 h with IV ofloxacin or ciprofloxacin and IV or oral doxycycline. *PID (ambulatory pt)*◇—**Adult:** 500 mg PO bid × 14 d (with 400 mg bid ofloxacin). Clostridium difficile *infect*◇—**Adult:** 750 mg/d to 2 g/d PO in three to four div doses × 7–14 d. Or, 500–750 mg IV q 6–8 h when PO dosing not feasible. Helicobacter pylori *related to peptic ulcer disease*◇—**Adult:** 250–500 mg PO tid to qid (with other drugs). Cont 7–14 d depending on regimen. **Child:** 15–20 mg/kg/d PO, div in two doses × 4 wk (with other drugs). *Amebiasis from* Dientamoeba fragilis◇—**Child:** 250 mg PO tid × 7 d. Entamoeba polecki *infect*◇—**Adult:** 750 mg PO tid × 10 d. **Child:** 35–50 mg/kg/d PO in three div doses × 10 d. *Dracunculiasis from* Dracunculus medinensis *(guinea worm infect)*◇—**Adult:** 250 mg PO tid × 10 d. **Child:** 25 mg/kg/d PO in three div doses (up to 750 mg/d) × 10 d. *Balantidiasis from* Balantidium coli◇—**Adult:** 750 mg PO tid × 5 d. **Child:** 35–50 mg/kg/d PO in three div doses × 5 d. *Symptomatic* Blastocystis hominis *infect*◇—**Adult:** 750 mg PO tid × 10 d. *Active Crohn's disease*◇—**Adult:** 400 mg PO bid. Refractory perineal disease,

20 mg/kg/d (1–1.5 g) in three to five div doses.
Prophx for sexual assault victim ◇ —**Adult:** 2 g PO with other drugs.

metronidazole (topical) • Flagyl, MetroCream, MetroGel, MetroGel-Vaginal, MetroLotion, Noritate

Nitroimidazole; antiprotozoal, antibacterial PRC: B	*Topical cream:* 0.75%, 1%; *Topical gel:* 0.75%; *Topical lotion:* 0.75%; *Vag gel:* 0.75%; *Tab:* 500 mg	*Topical tx of acne rosacea, pressure ulcer, inflammatory papules or pustules*—**Adult:** Thin film bid to affected area am and pm (once/d Noritate 1% topical gel). Significant results should occur within 3 wk and cont for first 9 wk of tx. *Topical tx of bacterial vaginosis*—**Adult:** One applicatorful vaginally, once/d or bid × 5 d or once at hs (nonpregnant). In low-risk pregnancy, one applicatorful vaginally bid × 5 d. *Tx of pressure ulcer* ◇ —**Adult:** Prepare 1% aqueous sol or susp from crushed sterilized tab; apply tid.

mezlocillin sodium • Mezlin

Extended-spectrum penicillin, acyclaminopenicillin; antibiotic PRC: B	*Inf:* 2 g, 3 g, 4 g; *Inj:* 1 g, 2 g, 3 g, 4 g	*Infect by susceptible organism*—**Adult:** 200–300 mg/kg/d IV or IM in four to six div doses. Usual dosage 3 g q 4 h or 4 g q 6 h. For serious infect, up to 24 g/d. Tx usually 10–14 d. **Child < 12 yr:** Mild to moderate infect, 50–100 mg/kg/d in four div doses. More severe infect, 200–300 mg/kg/d IM or IV in div doses q 4–6 h. **Neonate ≤ 7 d** ◇: 75 mg/kg q 12 h IV or IM. **Neonate ≥ 8 d:** 75 mg/kg q 8 h (if < 2 kg [4.4 lb]) or q 6 h (if > 2 kg) IV or IM. *Uncomplicated UTI*—**Adult:** 100–125 mg/kg/d IM or IV in div doses q 6 h or 1½–2 g q 6 h. *Complicated UTI*—**Adult:** 150–200 mg/kg/d IV div into q-6-h doses or 3 g q 6 h. *Uncomplicated gonococcal urethritis from* Neisseria gonorrhoeae—**Adult:** 1–2 g IM or IV with 1 g oral probenecid. *Surg prophx*—**Adult:** 4 g IV 30 min to 1½ h before surg; repeat IV 6 and 12 h later.

(continued)

Classes	Dosage Forms	Indications & Dosages
mezlocillin sodium *(continued)*		
		≡ ***Dosage adjustment.*** If CrCl 10–30 ml/min, give 3 g q 6–8 h for life-threatening or serious infect. For UTI, give 1.5 g q 6–8 h. If CrCl < 10 ml/min, give 2 g q 6–8 h for life-threatening or serious infect. For UTI, give 1.5 g q 8 h. Pts on hemodialysis should receive 3–4 g after each dialysis session; then q 12 h. Pts on peritoneal dialysis may receive 3 g q 12 h.
miconazole nitrate • Desenex, Femizol-M, Lotrimin AF, Micatin, Monistat-Derm, Monistat 3, Monistat 7, Monistat Dual-Pak		
Imidazole derivative; antifungal PRC: C	*Cream:* 1%, 2%; *Pwd:* 2%; *Spray:* 1%, 2%; *Topical oint:* 2%; *Topical sol:* 1%; *Vag cream:* 2%; *Vag supp:* 100 mg, 200 mg; *Kit:* 9 g 2% cream with seven 100-mg vag supp (Monistat 7); 9 g 2% cream with three 200-mg vag supp (Monistat 3); 9 g 2% cream with one 1,200-mg vag supp (Monistat Dual-Pak)	*Tinea corporis, tinea cruris, tinea pedis; cutaneous candidiasis; common dermatophyte infections*—**Adult, child > 1 yr:** Apply sparingly bid × 2–4 wk. Powder or spray can be used liberally on affected area. *Tinea versicolor*—**Adult, child > 1 yr:** Apply sparingly daily × 2 wk. *Vulvovaginal candidiasis*—**Adult:** 1 applicatorful or 100-mg supp (Monistat 7) vaginally hs × 7 d; repeat, if needed. Or, 200-mg supp (Monistat 3) vaginally hs × 3 d. Or, 1,200-mg supp (Monistat Dual-Pak) vaginally hs. Apply topical cream sparingly to affected area bid × 7 d.
minocycline hydrochloride • Dynacin, Minocin, Minocin IV, Vectrin		
Tetracycline derivative; antibiotic PRC: NR	*Caps:* 50 mg, 75 mg, 100 mg; *Inj:* 100 mg/vial; *Susp:* 50 mg/5 ml;	*Infect by sensitive organisms*—**Adult:** 200 mg PO, IV; then 100 mg q 12 h or 50 mg PO q 6 h. **Child > 8 yr:** 4 mg/kg PO, IV; then 4 mg/kg/d PO div q 12 h. Give IV in 500–1,000 ml sol without calcium, over 6 h.

Tab: 50 mg, 100 mg; *Ext-rel bioresorbable microspheres:* 1 mg per cartridge

Gonorrhea in pt sensitive to PCN—**Adult:** Initially, 200 mg PO; then 100 mg q 12 h × 4 d.
Syphilis in pt sensitive to PCN—**Adult:** 200 mg PO; then 100 mg q 12 h × 10–15 d.
Meningococcal carrier state—**Adult:** 200 mg PO; then 100 mg PO q 12 h × 5 d.
Uncomplicated urethral, endocervical, or rectal infection from Chlamydia trachomatis *or* Ureaplasma urealyticum—**Adult:** 100 mg PO q 12 h × ≥ 7 d.
Uncomplicated gonococcal urethritis—**Man:** 100 mg PO q 12 h × 5 d.
Infect with Mycobacterium marinum—**Adult:** 100 mg PO q 12 h × 6–8 wk.
Cholera—**Adult:** 200 mg PO; then 100 mg PO q 12 h × 72 h.
Acne—**Adult:** 50 mg/d PO daily to tid.
Multibacillary leprosy ◇ —**Adult:** 100 mg/d PO with clofazimine and ofloxacin × 6 mo; then 100 mg/d PO × 18 mo with clofazimine.
Nocardiosis ◇ —**Adult:** Usual dose × 12–18 mo.
Sclerosis agent for pleural effusion ◇ —**Adult:** 300 mg mixed in 40–50 ml sodium chloride inj by thoracostomy tube.
Nongonococcal urethritis from C. trachomatis *or* Mycoplasma pneumoniae ◇ —**Adult:** 100 mg/d PO in one or two div doses × 1–3 wk.
Adjunct tx of periodontitis—**Adult:** Place microspheres in infected periodontal pocket after scaling and planing.

moxifloxacin hydrochloride • Avelox, Avelox I.V.

Fluoroquinolone; antibiotic
PRC: C

Inf: 400 mg/250 ml; *Tab (film-coated):* 400 mg

Acute bacterial sinusitis from Haemophilus influenzae, Moraxella catarrhalis, Streptococcus pneumoniae—**Adult:** 400 mg PO or IV once/d × 10 d.
Acute bacterial exacer of chronic bronchitis from H. influenzae, H. parainfluenzae, Klebsiella pneumoniae, M. catarrhalis, Staphylococcus aureus, S. pneumoniae—**Adult:** 400 mg PO or IV once/d × 5 d.
Mild-to-moderate community-acquired pneumonia from Chlamydia pneumoniae, H. influenzae, M. catarrhalis, Mycoplasma pneumoniae, *(continued)*

Classes	Dosage Forms	Indications & Dosages
moxifloxacin hydrochloride *(continued)*		
		S. pneumoniae—**Adult:** 400 mg PO or IV once/d × 7–14 d. *Uncomplicated skin, skin-structure infect from* Staphylococcus aureus *or* S. pyogenes—**Adult:** 400 mg PO or IV once/d × 7 d.
mupirocin (pseudomonic acid A) • Bactroban **mupirocin calcium** • Bactroban Nasal		
Pseudomonic acid antibiotic; topical anti-infective PRC: B	*Cream:* 2%; *Oint:* 2% (1-g single-use tubes, 15 g, 30 g); *Oint (intranasal):* 2%	*Topical tx of impetigo from* Staphylococcus aureus, *beta-hemolytic* Streptococcus, Streptococcus pyogenes—**Adult, child:** Small amt to affected area tid × 1–2 wk. Cover with gauze dressing, if desired. *Eradication of nasal colonization of methicillin-resistant* S. aureus—**Adult:** Half of single-use tube to each nostril bid × 5 d. Press and release sides of nose repeatedly for 1 min to spread drug through nares.
nafcillin sodium • Nafcil, Nallpen, Unipen		
Penicillinase-resistant penicillin; antibiotic PRC: B	*Caps:* 250 mg; *Inj:* 500 mg, 1 g, 2 g; *IV inf piggyback:* 1 g, 2 g; *Pwd for oral sol:* 250 mg/ml (after reconst); *Tab:* 500 mg	*Systemic infect from susceptible organisms (methicillin-sensitive* Staphylococcus aureus)—**Adult:** 250–500 mg PO q 4–6 h for mild to moderate infect and 1 g q 4–6 h for more severe infect. Or, 500 mg IM q 4 h or 500–1,000 mg IV q 4 h based on severity of infect. **Child > 1 mo:** 50–100 mg/kg/d PO in div doses q 6 h. Or, 50–200 mg/kg/d IM or IV in div doses q 4–6 h based on severity of infect. **Neonate:** 30–40 mg/kg/d PO div equally into three to four doses. Or, 20 mg/kg/d IM div in two equal doses. Or, if < 7 d old, 40 mg/kg/d IM div in two equal doses q 12 h; if 7–28 d old, 60–200 mg/kg/d in div doses q 8 h. For mild-to-moderate infect, may give 50–100 mg/kg/d IV in div doses q 6 h. For more severe infect, 100–200 mg/kg/d IV div q 4–6 h. Or, 25 mg/kg IV q 12 h (if < 7 d old and < 2 kg) or q 8 h (if < 7 d old and > 2 kg or > 7 d old and < 2 kg) or q 6 h (if > 7 d old and > 2 kg).

Meningitis—**Neonate < 7 d and weighing < 2 kg:** 50 mg/kg IV q 12 h. **Neonate < 7 d and weighing > 2 kg:** 50 mg/kg IV q 8 h. **Neonate > 7 d and weighing < 2 kg:** 50 mg/kg IV q 8 h. **Neonate > 7 d and > 2 kg:** 50 mg/kg IV q 6 h.
Acute or chronic osteomyelitis from susceptible organism—**Adult:** 1–2 g IV q 4 h × 4–8 wk.
Meningitis from susceptible organism—**Adult:** 100–200 mg/kg/d IV in div doses q 4–6 h.
Native valve endocarditis from susceptible organism—**Adult:** 2 g IV q 4 h × 4–6 wk with gentamicin.

nalidixic acid • NegGram

Quinolone antibiotic; urinary tract anti-infective
PRC: B

Susp: 250 mg/5 ml; *Tab:* 250 mg, 500 mg, 1 g

Acute and chronic UTI from susceptible gram-negative organism—**Adult:** 1 g PO qid × 7–14 d; 2 g/d PO for long-term use. Up to 6 g/d for severe UTI. **Child > 3 mo:** 55 mg/kg/d PO div qid × 7–14 d; 33 mg/kg/d PO div qid for long-term use.

nelfinavir mesylate • Viracept

HIV protease inhibitor; antiviral
PRC: B

Pwd: 50 mg/g; *Tab:* 250 mg

HIV infect when antiretroviral tx warranted—**Adult:** 750 mg PO tid with meal or light snack. **Child 2–13 yr:** 20–30 mg/kg/dose PO tid with meal or light snack. Max, 750 mg tid. Recommended ped dosage tid as follows: If pt weighs 7–8.4 kg, four 1-g scoops or 1 level tsp; if 8.5–10.4 kg, five 1-g scoops or 1.25 level tsp; if 10.5–11.9 kg, six 1-g scoops or 1.5 level tsp; if 12–13.9 kg, seven 1-g scoops or 1.75 level tsp; if 14–15.9 kg, eight 1-g scoops or 2 level tsp; if 16–17.9 kg, nine 1-g scoops or 2.25 level tsp; if 18–22.9 kg, 10 1-g scoops or 2.5 level tsp or 2 tab; if ≥ 23 kg, 15 1-g scoops or 3.75 level tsp or 3 tab. **Child 2–13 yr and weighing 23–53 kg** ◇: 25–30 mg/kg PO tid to 1,250 or 1,500 mg/dose.
Prophx after occupational exposure to HIV ◇—**Adult:** 750 mg PO tid with oral zidovudine and lamivudine × 4 wk.

Classes	Dosage Forms	Indications & Dosages
neomycin sulfate • Mycifradin, Myciguent, Neo-fradin, Neo-Tabs		
Aminoglycoside; antibiotic PRC: D	**Rx only:** *Oral sol:* 125 mg/5 ml; *Otic susp:* 5 mg/ml (with polymyxin B sulfate 10,000 units/ml and hydrocortisone 1%); *Tab:* 500 mg **OTC:** *Cream:* 0.5%; *Oint:* 0.5%	*Infectious diarrhea from enteropathogenic* Escherichia coli—**Adult:** 50 mg/kg/d PO in four div doses × 2–3 d. **Child:** 50–100 mg/kg/d PO div q 4–6 h × 2–3 d. *Suppression of intestinal bacteria preop*—**Adult:** 1 g PO q 1 h × four doses; then 1 g q 4 h for rest of 24 h. Saline cathartic precedes tx. **Child:** 40–100 mg/kg/d PO div q 4–6 h. Precede first dose with saline cathartic. For 2–3 d regimen, 88 mg/kg PO in six equal div doses at 4-h intervals. Or, for 8 am surg, 1 g neomycin and 1 g erythromycin base PO at 1 pm, 2 pm, and 11 pm day before surg. *Adjunct tx in hepatic coma*—**Adult:** 1–3 g PO qid × 5–6 d; 200 ml of 1% or 100 ml of 2% sol as enema retained 20–60 min q 6 h. **Child:** 50–100 mg/kg/d PO in div doses × 5–6 d. *Hypercholesterolemia* ◊ —**Adult:** 500 mg/d to 2 g/d PO in two or three div doses. *External ear canal infect*—**Adult, child:** 2–5 gtt into ear canal tid or qid × 7–10 d. *Topical bacterial infect, burn, wound, skin graft, surg, lesions, pruritus, trophic ulcerations, edema*—**Adult, child:** Rub in small amt gently bid, tid, or as directed. ≡ ***Dosage adjustment.*** Reduce dosage in adults and children with renal impairment.
nevirapine • Viramune		
Nonnucleoside reverse transcriptase inhibitor; antiviral	*Oral susp:* 50 mg/5 ml; *Tab:* 200 mg	*HIV-1 infect (with other antiretrovirals)*—**Adult, adolescent:** 200 mg/d PO × 14 d; then 200 mg PO q 12 h. **Child 2 mo–8 yr:** 4 mg/kg PO once/d × 14 d; then 7 mg/kg PO q 12 h. Max, 400 mg/d. **Child ≥ 8 yr:** 4 mg/kg PO once/d ×

PRC: C

14 d; then 4 mg/kg PO q 12 h. Max, 400 mg/d. Or, 120 mg/m²/d PO × 14 d; then 120–200 mg/m² q 12 h. **Neonate** ◇: 5 mg/kg/d PO × 14 d; then 120 mg/m² q 12 h × next 14 d; then 200 mg/m² q 12 h.

nitrofurantoin macrocrystals • Macrobid, Macrodantin
nitrofurantoin microcrystals • Furadantin

Nitrofuran; urinary tract anti-infective
PRC: B

macrocrystals *Caps:* 25 mg, 50 mg, 100 mg; *Caps (dual-rel):* 100 mg; **microcrystals** *Susp:* 25 mg/5 ml

Initial or recurrent UTI from susceptible organism—**Adult, child > 12 yr:** 50–100 mg PO qid or 100 mg dual-rel caps q 12 h × 7 d. **Child 1 mo–12 yr:** 5–7 mg/kg/d PO in four div doses.
Long-term suppression tx—**Adult:** 50–100 mg/d PO hs single dose. **Child:** Low as 1 mg/kg/d PO single dose or two div doses.

nitrofurazone • Furacin

Nitrofuran derivative; synthetic antibacterial
PRC: C

Cream: 0.2%; *Oint:* 0.2% (soluble dressing); *Topical sol:* 0.2%

Adjunct tx of second- and third-degree burns (especially with resistance to other antibiotics and sulfonamides), prophx of allograft rejection—**Adult, child:** Apply to lesion daily or q few d based on severity of burn. May also be applied to dressings covering affected area.

norfloxacin (ophthalmic) • Chibroxin

Fluoroquinolone; broad-spectrum antibiotic
PRC: C

Ophth sol: 0.3% in 5-ml containers

Conjunctivitis from susceptible organism—**Adult, child ≥ 1 yr:** 1–2 gtt in affected eye qid × up to 7 d. If needed, 1–2 gtt may be applied q 2 h while awake on first 1–2 d of tx.

norfloxacin (systemic) • Noroxin

Fluoroquinolone; broad-spectrum antibiotic
PRC: C

Tab: 400 mg

Complicated and uncomplicated UTI from certain gram-neg and gram-pos bacteria—**Adult:** For complicated infect, 400 mg PO bid × 10–21 d. For uncomplicated infect, 400 mg PO bid × 3–10 d. Max, 800 mg/d.
Uncomplicated gonorrhea—**Adult:** 800 mg PO single dose.
Prostatitis—**Adult:** 400 mg PO q 12 h × 28 d.

(continued)

Classes	Dosage Forms	Indications & Dosages
norfloxacin (systemic) *(continued)*		
		Gastroenteritis ◇ —**Adult:** 400 mg PO bid × 5 d. *Traveler's diarrhea* ◇ —**Adult:** 400 mg PO bid × up to 3 d. ≡ ***Dosage adjustment.*** If CrCl < 30 ml/min, give 400 mg/d for duration of tx.
nystatin • Mycostatin, Nadostine ♦, Nilstat, Nystex		
Polyene macrolide; antifungal PRC: C	*Cream:* 100,000 units/g; *Lozenges:* 200,000 units; *Oint:* 100,000 units/g; *Pwd:* 100,000 units/g; *Pwd for susp:* 50-, 150-, 500-million units; 1-, 2-, 5-billion units; *Susp:* 100,000 units/ml; *Tab:* 500,000 units; *Vag supp:* 100,000 units	*Oropharyngeal candidiasis*—**Adult, child:** 400,000–600,000 units oral susp qid. Or, 200,000–400,000 units (lozenges) four to five times/d × up to 14 d (dissolved in mouth). **Infant:** 200,000 units oral susp qid. **Neonate, premature infant:** 100,000 units oral susp qid. *Oropharyngeal candidiasis in HIV infect*—**Adult:** 500,000–1,000,000 units three to five times/d as oral susp or tab (dissolved in mouth). Or, oral lozenges may be used. *Cutaneous or mucocutaneous candidal infect*—**Topical use:** Apply to affected areas bid or tid until healing complete (about 2 wk). **Vag use:** Insert vag supp high into vagina daily or bid × 14 d. *Prophx of thrush*—**Neonate:** 100,000- to 200,000-unit vag tab daily × 3–6 wk before delivery. *Candidal diaper dermatitis*—**Infant:** 100,000 units oral susp PO qid as adjunct to topical nystatin. *GI infect*—**Adult:** 500,000–1 million units as PO tab, tid.
ofloxacin 0.3% (ophth) • Ocuflox		
Fluoroquinolone; antibiotic PRC: C	*Ophth sol:* 0.3% in 1-ml and 5-ml solution	*Conjunctivitis from* Staphylococcus aureus, S. epidermidis, Streptococcus pneumoniae, Enterobacter cloacae, Haemophilus influenzae, Proteus mirabilis, Pseudomonas aeruginosa, Propionibacterium acnes—**Adult, child > 1 yr:** 1–2 gtt in conjunctival sac q 2–4 h while awake × 2 d; then qid × up to 5 more d.

		Bacterial corneal ulcer from S. aureus, S. epidermidis, S. pneumoniae, E. cloacae, H. influenzae, P. mirabilis, P. aeruginosa, Serratia marcescens, P. acnes—**Adult, child > 1 yr:** 1–2 gtt q 30 min while awake and 1–2 gtt 4–6 h after retiring on d 1 and 2. D 3–7, 1–2 gtt/h while awake. D 7–9, 1–2 gtt qid.

ofloxacin 0.3% (otic) • Floxin Otic

Fluoroquinolone; antibiotic PRC: C	*Otic sol:* 0.3%	*Otitis externa*—**Adult, child > 12 yr:** 10 gtt in affected ear bid × 10 d. **Child 1–12 yr:** 5 gtt in affected ear bid × 10 d. *Acute otitis media in pts with tympanostomy tubes*—**Child 1–12 yr:** 5 gtt in affected ear bid × 10 d. *Chronic suppurative otitis media with perforated tympanic membrane*—**Adult, child ≥ 12 yr:** 10 gtt in affected ear bid × 14 d.

ofloxacin (systemic) • Floxin, Floxin I.V.

Fluoroquinolone; antibiotic PRC: C	*Inj:* 200 mg in 50 ml D_5W; 400 mg in water for inj in 10-ml single-use vials; 400 mg in 100 ml D_5W; *Tab:* 200 mg, 300 mg, 400 mg	*Acute bacterial exacer of chronic bronchitis and pneumonia from susceptible organism; mild-to-moderate skin, skin-structure infect; community-acquired pneumonia*—**Adult:** 400 mg PO or IV q 12 h × 10 d. *Sexually transmitted diseases, such as acute uncomplicated urethral and cervical gonorrhea, nongonococcal urethritis and cervicitis, and mixed infect of urethra and cervix*—**Adult:** Acute uncomplicated gonorrhea, 400 mg PO or IV once as single dose; cervicitis and urethritis, 300 mg PO or IV q 12 h × 7 d. *UTI*—**Adult:** Cystitis from *Escherichia coli* or *Klebsiella pneumoniae,* 200 mg PO or IV q 12 h × 3 d; cystitis from other organisms, 200 mg PO or IV q 12 h × 7 d. *Complicated UTI*—**Adult:** 400 mg PO or IV q 12 h × 10 d. *Prostatitis*—**Adult:** 300 mg PO or IV q 12 h × ≥ 6 wk. Change from IV to PO after 10 d. *PID*—**Adult:** 400 mg PO q 12 h with metronidazole × 14 d. Or, 400 mg IV q 12 h with metronidazole × 10–14 d.

(continued)

Classes	Dosage Forms	Indications & Dosages
ofloxacin (systemic) *(continued)*		
		Adjunct in Brucella *infect* ◇ —**Adult:** 400 mg/d PO × 6 wk. *Peritonitis in pt receiving continuous ambulatory peritoneal dialysis* ◇ —**Adult:** 400 mg PO loading dose; then 300 mg/d PO × 7–10 d. *Antituberculosis agent (adjunct)* ◇ —**Adult:** 300 mg/d PO. *Postop sternotomy or soft-tissue wound from* Mycobacterium fortuitum ◇—**Adult:** 300 or 600 mg/d PO once/d × 3–6 mo. *Acute Q fever pneumonia from* Coxiella burnetii ◇ —**Adult:** 600 mg/d PO × ≤ 16 d. *Traveler's diarrhea* ◇ —**Adult:** 300 mg PO bid × 3 d. *Lower respiratory tract or skin infect*—**Adult:** 200–400 mg PO q 12 h × 10 d. ≡ ***Dosage adjustment.*** If CrCl 10–50 ml/min, give initial dose as recommended and then usual PO dose q 24 h. If CrCl < 10 ml/min, give recommended initial dose and then half of usual PO dose q 24 h.
oseltamivir phosphate • Tamiflu		
Influenza virus neuraminidase inhibitor; antiviral PRC: C	*Caps:* 75 mg; *Susp:* 12 mg/ml	*Uncomplicated, acute influenza A and B infect in pt with symptoms ≤ 2 d*—**Adult:** 75 mg PO twice bid × 5 d, starting ≤ 2 d of symptom onset. ≡ ***Dosage adjustment.*** For adult with CrCl < 30 ml/min, 75 mg PO once/d × 5 d, starting ≤ 2 d of symptom onset. *Influenza in child ≤ 1 yr*—**Child weighing ≤ 15 kg:** 30 mg oral susp PO bid. **Child 15–23 kg:** 45 mg oral susp PO bid. **Child weighing 23–40 kg:** 60 mg oral susp PO bid. **Child weighing > 40 kg:** 75 mg oral susp PO bid. *Prophx of influenza after close contact with infected person*—**Adult, adolescent ≤ 13 yr:** 75 mg PO once/d starting ≤ 2 d after exposure and lasting ≤ 7 d. *Prophx of influenza during community outbreak*—**Adult, adolescent ≤ 13 yr:** 75 mg PO once/d up to 6 wk.

≡ ***Dosage adjustment.*** If CrCl < 30 ml/min, 75 mg PO every other d × 5 d, starting ≤ 2 d of exposure.

oxacillin sodium • Bactocill

Penicillinase-resistant PCN; antibiotic PRC: B	*Caps:* 250 mg, 500 mg; *Inj:* 250 mg, 500 mg, 1 g, 2 g, 4 g; *IV inf:* 1 g, 2 g, 4 g; *Oral sol:* 250 mg/5 ml (after reconst)	*Systemic infect from* Staphylococcus aureus—**Adult, child weighing > 40 kg:** 500 mg PO q 4–6 h for mild-to-moderate infect. When changing from IV to PO, 1 g PO q 4–6 h. Or, 250–500 mg IM or IV q 4–6 h. For more severe infect, 1 g or more IV or IM q 4–6 h. Serious infect treated × 1–2 wk. **Child > 1 mo and weighing < 40 kg:** 50–100 mg/kg/d PO div and given q 4–6 h. Or, 50–200 mg/kg/d IM or IV, div and given q 4–6 h. Doses vary with severity of infect. *Acute or chronic osteomyelitis from susceptible organism*—**Adult:** 1.5–2 g IV q 4 h × 4–8 wk or IV dose × 5–28 d followed by PO dose × 3–6 wk for total of 6 wk tx. *Native valve endocarditis caused by methicillin-susceptible staphylococci*—**Adult:** 2 g IV q 4 h × 4–6 wk with gentamicin for first 3–5 d. *Prosthetic valve endocarditis from methicillin-susceptible staphylococci*—**Adult:** 2 g IV q 4 h × ≥ 6 wk with gentamicin and rifampin. ≡ ***Dosage adjustment.*** If adult's CrCl < 10 ml/min, 1 g IM or IV q 4–6 h.

palivizumab • Synagis

Recombinant monoclonal antibody IgG1$_K$; respiratory syncytial virus (RSV) prophx PRC: C	*Inj:* 50-mg, 100-mg single-use vial	*Prophx of serious lower respiratory tract disease from RSV in child at high risk*—**Child:** 15 mg/kg/mo IM throughout RSV season. Give first dose before RSV season.

Classes	Dosage Forms	Indications & Dosages
penicillin G benzathine • Bicillin L-A, Permapen **penicillin G benzathine and procaine** • Bicillin C-R **penicillin G potassium** • Pfizerpen **penicillin G procaine** • Ayercillin ◆, Bicillin C-R, Wycillin **penicillin G sodium**		
Natural PCN; antibiotic PRC: B	**PCN G benzathine** *Inj:* 300,000 units/ml; 600,000 units/ml; 1.2 million units/2 ml; 2.4 million units/4 ml; *Susp:* 250,000 units/5ml ◆; 500,000 units/ml ◆; **PCN G benzathine and procaine** *Inj:* 300,000 units/ml; 600,000 units/ml; **PCN G potassium** *Inj (premixed, frozen):* 1 million units/50 ml, 2 million units/50 ml, 3 million units/50 ml; *Pwd for inj:* 1 million units, 5 million units, 10 million units, 20 million units; **PCN G procaine** *Inj:* 600,000 units/ml; **PCN G**	*Congenital syphilis (PCN G benzathine)*—**Child < 2 yr:** 50,000 units/kg IM as single inj. *Group A streptococcal upper respiratory infections, diphtheria, yaws, pinta, bejel (PCN G benzathine)*—**Adult:** 1.2 million units IM as single inj. **Child weighing ≥ 27 kg:** 900,000 units IM as single inj. **Child weighing < 27 kg:** 300,000–600,000 units IM as single inj. *Prophx of poststreptococcal rheumatic fever (PCN G benzathine)*—**Adult, child:** 1.2 million units IM once/mo. *Syphilis < 1 yr duration (PCN G benzathine)*—**Adult:** 2.4 million units IM as single dose. *Syphilis > 1 yr duration (PCN G benzathine)*—**Adult:** 2.4 million units/wk IM × 3 wk. *Moderate-to-severe systemic infect (PCN G potassium, sodium)*—**Adult:** 12–24 million units/d IM or IV in div doses q 4 h. **Child:** 25,000–300,000 units/kg/d IM or IV in div doses q 4 h. *Moderate-to-severe systemic infect, pneumococcal pneumonia (PCN G procaine)*—**Adult:** 600,000–1.2 million units/d IM as single dose or q 6–12 h. **Child:** 300,000 units/d IM as single dose. *Uncomplicated gonorrhea (PCN G procaine)*—**Adult, child > 12 yr:** 1 g probenecid PO; then, 30 min later, 4.8 million units PCN G procaine IM, divided into two inj sites.

	sodium *Pwd for inj:* 1 million units ◆, 5 million units, 10 million units ◆	*Anthrax (PCN G potassium)*—**Adult:** 5–20 million units/d IV in div doses q 4–6 h × ≥ 14 d after symptoms abate. Or, 80,000 units/kg in first hour; then maint dose of 320,000 units/kg/d. Average adult dose is 4 million units q 4 h; can also be given as 2 million units q 2 h. **Child:** 100,000–250,000 units/kg/d IV in div doses q 4–6 h × ≥ 14 d after symptoms abate. *Anthrax from* Bacillus anthracis, *including inhal anthrax post-exposure (PCN G procaine)*—**Adult:** 1.2 million units IM q 12 h. **Child:** 25,000 units/kg IM (max, 1.2 million units) q 12 h. *Cutaneous anthrax (PCN G procaine)*—**Adult:** 600,000–1 million units/d IM. ≡ ***Dosage adjustment.*** If CrCl 10–50 ml/min, give half usual dose q 4–5 h or usual dose q 8–12 h. If CrCl < 10 ml/min, give half usual dose q 8–12 h or usual dose q 12–18 h.

penicillin V potassium • Apo-Pen-VK ◆, Beepen-VK, Betapen-VK, Nadopen-V ◆, Novo-Pen VK ◆, Nu-Pen-VK ◆, Pen Vee K, Penicillin VK, PVF K ◆, V-Cillin K, Veetids

Natural PCN; antibiotic PRC: B	*Sol:* 125 mg/5 ml, 250 mg/5 ml (after reconst); *Tab:* 250 mg, 500 mg; *Tab (film-coated):* 250 mg, 500 mg	*Mild-to-moderate susceptible infect*—**Adult, child ≥ 12 yr:** 125–500 mg (200,000–800,000 units) PO q 6 h. **Child 1 mo–12 yr:** 15–62.5 mg/kg/d PO div and given q 6–8 h. *Necrotizing ulcerative gingivitis*—**Adult:** 250–500 mg PO q 6–8 h. *Lyme disease* ◇ —**Adult:** 250–500 mg PO qid × 10–20 d. *Prophx for pneumococcal infect* ◇ —**Adult:** 250 mg PO bid. **Child > 5 yr:** 125 mg PO bid. *Prophx for rheumatic fever*—**Adult, child ≥ 12 yr:** 250 mg PO bid.

piperacillin sodium • Pipracil

Extended-spectrum PCN; acylamino-penicillin antibiotic	*Inf:* 2 g, 3 g, 4 g; *Inj:* 2 g, 3 g, 4 g	*Infect from susceptible organism*—**Adult, child > 12 yr:** For serious infect, 12–18 g/d IV in div doses q 4–6 h. For uncomplicated UTI and community-acquired pneumonia, 6–8 g/d IV in div doses q 6–12 h. *(continued)*

Classes	Dosage Forms	Indications & Dosages
piperacillin sodium *(continued)*		
PRC: B		For complicated UTI, 8–16 g/d IV in div doses q 6–8 h. For uncomplicated gonorrhea, 2 g IM as single dose. Max, 24 g/d. **Child 1 mo–12 yr:** 50 mg/kg IV over 30 min q 4 h. *Prophx of surg infect*—**Adult:** For intra-abdominal surg, 2 g IV before surg, 2 g during surg, and 2 g q 6 h after surg × ≤ 24 h. For vag hysterectomy, 2 g IV before surg, 2 g 6 h after first dose, and 2 g 12 h after second dose. For cesarean section, 2 g IV after cord clamped; then 2 g q 4 h × two doses. For abdominal hysterectomy, 2 g IV before surg, 2 g in postanesthesia care unit, and 2 g after 6 h. ≡ ***Dosage adjustment.*** If CrCl 20–40 ml/min, give 3 g q 8 h for complicated UTI and 4 g q 8 h for serious systemic infect. If CrCl < 20 ml/min, give 3 g q 12 h for uncomplicated or complicated UTI and 4 g q 12 h for serious systemic infect.
piperacillin sodium and tazobactam sodium • Zosyn		
Extended-spectrum PCN and beta-lactamase inhibitor; antibiotic PRC: B	*Pwd for inj (equivalent to piperacillin/tazobactam in ratio of 8:1):* 2.25 g, 3.375 g, 4.5 g	*Moderate-to-severe infect from piperacillin-resistant, piperacillin/tazobactam-susceptible, beta-lactamase–producing strains of microorganisms in these conditions: appendicitis (complicated by rupture or abscess) and peritonitis from* Escherichia coli, Bacteroides fragilis, B. ovatus, B. thetaiotaomicron, B. vulgatus; *skin, skin-structure infect from* Staphylococcus aureus; *postpartum endometritis or PID from* E. coli; *moderately severe community-acquired pneumonia from* Haemophilus influenzae—**Adult:** 3.375 g (3 g piperacillin/0.375 g tazobactam) q 6 h as 30-min IV inf. ≡ ***Dosage adjustment.*** If adult or child > 12 has CrCl 20–40 ml/min, give 2.25 g (2 g piperacillin/0.25 g tazobactam) q 6 h. If CrCl < 20 ml/min, give

2.25 g (2 g piperacillin/0.25 g tazobactam) q 8 h. If pt receives hemodialysis, give 2.25 g (2 g piperacillin/0.25 g tazobactam) q 8 h with suppl dose of 0.75 g (0.67 g piperacillin/0.09 g tazobactam) after each session.

polymyxin B sulfate • Polymyxin B sulfate

Polymyxin; antibiotic PRC: C	*Ophth sterile pwd for sol:* 500,000-unit vials reconst to 20–50 ml	*Superficial eye infect from* Pseudomonas *or other gram-neg organism involving conjunctiva and cornea (alone or with other drugs)*—**Adult, child:** 1–3 gtt of 0.1%–0.25% (10,000–25,000 units/ml) hourly. Increase interval based on pt response. Max for adult, 10,000 units/d by subconjunctival inj or 2 million units/d or 25,000 units/kg/d if applied topically.

primaquine phosphate • primaquine phosphate

8-aminoquinoline; antimalarial PRC: C	*Tab:* 26.3 mg (15-mg base); *Pwd:* 5, 25, 100 g	*Radical cure of relapsing vivax malaria, eliminating symptoms and infect completely, and prophx of relapse*—**Adult:** 15 mg/d (base) PO × 14 d (26.3-mg tab = 15 mg base) or 79 mg (45-mg base) PO once/wk × 8 wk. **Child:** 0.3 mg/kg/d (base) PO × 14 d. Pneumocystis carinii *pneumonia* ◇ —**Adult:** 15–30 mg/d (base) PO.

pyrazinamide • pms-Pyrazinamide ♦, Tebrazid ♦

Synthetic pyrazine analogue of nicotinamide; antituberculotic PRC: C	*Tab:* 500 mg	*Adjunct TB tx when primary and secondary antituberculotics can't be used or have failed*—**Adult:** 15–30 mg/kg/d PO in one or more doses. Max, 2 g/d. Or a twice/wk dose of 50–70 mg/kg (based on lean body weight) to promote pt compliance; dosages above 3 g twice/wk have been well tolerated. ≡ ***Dosage adjustment.*** Select low-end dosage if pt has renal impairment. Discontinue if any signs of hepatic injury occur.

Classes	Dosage Forms	Indications & Dosages
pyrimethamine • Daraprim **pyrimethamine with sulfadoxine** • Fansidar		
Folic acid antagonist; antimalarial PRC: C	**pyrimethamine** *Tab:* 25 mg; **pyrimethamine with sulfadoxine** *Tab:* pyrimethamine 25 mg, sulfadoxine 500 mg	*Malaria prophx and transmission control (pyrimethamine)*—**Adult, child ≥ 10 yr:** 25 mg/wk PO × 6–10 wk or more after leaving malaria-endemic area. **Child 4–10 yr:** 12.5 mg/wk PO cont × 6–10 wk or more after leaving malaria-endemic area. **Child < 4 yr:** 6.25 mg/wk PO cont × 6–10 wk or more after leaving endemic area. *Malaria prophx and transmission control (pyrimethamine with sulfadoxine)*—**Adult, child ≥ 14 yr:** 1 tab/wk or 2 tab q 2 wk during exposure and × 4–6 wk afterward. **Child 9–14 yr:** ¾ tab/wk or 1½ tab q 2 wk during exposure and × 4–6 wk afterward. **Child 4–8 yr:** ½ tab/wk or 1 tab q 2 wk during exposure and × 4–6 wk afterward. **Child < 4 yr:** ¼ tab/wk or ½ tab q 2 wk during exposure and × 4–6 wk afterward. *Acute malaria attack (pyrimethamine)*—**Adult:** 50 mg/d PO × 2 d; then 25 mg once/wk × ≥ 10 wk. **Child 4–10 yr:** 25 mg PO once/d × 2 d; then 12.5 mg once/wk × ≥ 10 wk. *Acute malaria attack (pyrimethamine with sulfadoxine)*—Given on last day of quinine tx. **Adult, child ≥ 14 yr:** 3 tab as single dose. **Child 9–14 yr:** 2 tab as single dose. **Child 4–8 yr:** 1 tab as single dose. **Child 1–3 yr:** ½ tab as single dose. **Child 2–11 mo:** ¼ tab as single dose. *Toxoplasmosis (pyrimethamine)*—**Adult:** 50–75 mg PO with 1–4 g sulfadiazine; cont 1–3 wk. After 3 wk, reduce dosage by half and cont 4–5 wk. **Child:** 1 mg/kg/d PO in two equal div doses × 2–4 d; then 0.5 mg/kg/d × 4 wk with 100 mg sulfadiazine/kg/d PO, div q 6 h. Max, 100 mg.

quinupristin and dalfopristin • Synercid

Streptogramin; antibiotic PRC: B	*Inj:* 500 mg/10 ml (150 mg quinupristin and 350 mg dalfopristin)	*Serious or life-threatening infect from vancomycin-resistant* Enterococcus faecium *bacteremia*—**Adult, adolescent ≥ 16 yr:** 7.5 mg/kg by IV inf over 1 h q 8 h. Duration determined by site and severity of infect. *Complicated skin, skin-structure infect from* Staphylococcus aureus *(methicillin susceptible),* Streptococcus pyogenes—**Adult, adolescent ≥ 16 yr:** 7.5 mg/kg by IV inf over 1 h q 12 h × ≥ 7 d.

ribavirin • Virazole

Synthetic nucleoside; antiviral PRC: X	*Pwd to be reconst for inhal:* 6 g in 100-ml glass vial	*Tx of hospitalized infant or young child with respiratory syncytial virus (RSV) infect*—**Infant, young child:** 20-mg/ml sol via Viratek Small Particle Aerosol Generator (SPAG-2) to make mist of 190 mcg/L. Tx cont 12–18 h/d × ≥ 3 and < 7 d with flow rate of 12.5 L mist/min. For ventilated pt, use same dose with pressure- or volume-cycled ventilator and SPAG-2. Suction pt q 1–2 h and check pulmonary pressures q 2–4 h.

rifabutin • Mycobutin

Semisynthetic ansamycin; antibiotic, antituberculotic PRC: B	*Caps:* 150 mg	*Primary prev of disseminated MAC in pts with advanced HIV infect*—**Adult:** 300 mg/d PO single dose or div bid with food. *Active TB*◇—**Adult not receiving antiretroviral tx:** First phase (2 wk–2 mo): 5 mg/kg/d (max, 300 mg) with isoniazid 5 mg/kg/d (max, 300 mg), ethambutol 15–25 mg/kg/d (max, 1.6 g), and pyrazinamide 15–30 mg/kg/d (max, 2 g). Second phase: 5 mg/kg/d (max, 300 mg) or twice/wk with isoniazid 5 mg/kg/d max, 300 mg) or 15 mg/kg (max, 900 mg) twice/wk × ≥ 4 mo. **Child not receiving antiretroviral tx:** First phase (2 wk–2 mo): 10–20 mg/kg/d (max, 300 mg) with isoniazid 10–20 mg/kg/d (max, 300 mg), ethambutol 15–25 mg/kg/d (max, 1.6 g), and pyrazinamide 15–30 mg/kg/d *(conbtinued)*

Classes	Dosage Forms	Indications & Dosages
rifabutin *(conbtinued)*		
		(max, 2 g). Second phase: 10–20 mg/kg/d (max, 300 mg) or twice/wk with isoniazid 10–20 mg/kg/d (max, 300 mg) or 20–40 mg/kg (max, 900 mg) twice/wk × ≥ 4 mo.
rifampin • Rifadin, Rimactane		
Semisynthetic rifamycin B derivative (macrocyclic antibiotic); antituberculotic PRC: C	*Caps:* 150 mg, 300 mg; *Inj:* 600 mg/vial	*Primary tx in pulmonary TB*—**Adult:** 600 mg/d PO or IV as single dose. Give PO dose 1 h before or 2 h after meal. **Child:** 10–20 mg/kg/d PO or IV single dose. Give PO dose 1 h before or 2 h after meal. Max, 600 mg/d. Concurrent use of other antituberculotic recommended. Tx usually lasts 6–9 mo. *Asymptomatic meningococcal carrier*—**Adult:** 600 mg PO bid × 2 d. **Infant, child > 1 mo:** 10 mg/kg PO bid × 2 d. **Neonate < 1 mo:** 5 mg/kg PO bid × 2 d. *Prev of infect from* Haemophilus influenzae *type B*—**Adult, child:** 20 mg/kg (up to 600 mg) once/d × 4 d. *Leprosy*◇—**Adult:** 600 mg PO once/mo, usually with other drugs.
rifapentine • Priftin		
Cyclopentyl rifamycin; antibiotic PRC: C	*Tab (film-coated):* 150 mg	*Pulmonary TB, with at least one other antituberculotic to which isolate is susceptible*—**Adult:** During intensive phase of short-course therapy, 600 mg PO twice/wk × 2 mo, with ≥ 72 h between doses. During continuation phase of short-course therapy, 600 mg PO once/wk × 4 mo with isoniazid or another drug.
rimantadine hydrochloride • Flumadine		
Synthetic amantadine derivative; antiviral	*Syrup:* 50 mg/5 ml; *Tab:* 100 mg	*Prophx for influenza A virus*—**Adult, child ≥ 10 yr:** 100 mg PO bid. **Child < 10 yr:** 5 mg/kg PO once/d. Max dose, 150 mg.

PRC: C

Tx of illness from influenza A virus—**Adult:** 100 mg PO bid × 7 d from symptom onset. **Elderly pt in communal setting:** 100 mg/d PO.

≡ ***Dosage adjustment.*** In severe hepatic or renal impairment (CrCl ≤ 10 ml/min) and for elderly pts in communal settings, reduce to 100 mg/d PO.

ritonavir • Norvir

HIV protease inhibitor; antiviral
PRC: B

Caps: 100 mg; *Oral sol:* 80 mg/ml

HIV infect when antiretroviral tx warranted—**Adult:** 600 mg PO bid with meals. If nausea occurs: 300 mg bid, incr q 2–3 d by 100 mg bid, up to 600 mg bid. **Child ≥ 2 yr:** 400 mg/m^2 PO bid with other antiretrovirals. To minimize nausea, initially 250 mg/m^2 bid and incr by 50 mg/m^2 bid q 2–3 d.

saquinavir • Fortovase
saquinavir mesylate • Invirase

HIV-1 and HIV-2 proteinase inhibitor; antiviral
PRC: B

saquinavir *Caps (soft gelatin):* 200 mg; **saquinavir mesylate** *Caps (hard gelatin):* 200 mg

Adjunct tx of advanced HIV infect in selected pts—**Adult:** 600 mg (Invirase, three 200-mg caps) PO tid within 2 h after full meal with nucleoside analogue. Or, 1,200 mg (Fortovase, six 200-mg caps) tid within 2 h after full meal with nucleoside analogue.

silver nitrate • Silver Nitrate

Heavy metal (silver compound); ophth antiseptic, topical cauterizing
PRC: C

Ophth sol: 1%; *Topical oint:* 10%; *Topical sol:* 10%, 25%, 50%

Prev of gonorrheal ophthalmia neonatorum—**Neonate:** Clean lids thoroughly; instill 2 gtt 1% sol in lower conjunctival sac each eye; ensure sol has contact with entire conjunctival sac ≥ 30 sec.

To treat indolent wounds, destroy exuberant granulations, freshen edges of ulcers and fissures, provide styptic action, treat vesicular bullous or aphthous lesions—**Adult:** Apply oint (on pad) to lesion × 5 d. Or, cotton applicator dipped in sol to affected area two to three times/wk × 2–3 wk.

Classes	Dosage Forms	Indications & Dosages
sparfloxacin • Zagam		
Fluorinated quinolone; broad-spectrum antibacterial PRC: C	*Tab:* 200 mg	*Acute bacterial exacer of chronic bronchitis from* Staphylococcus aureus, Streptococcus pneumoniae, Chlamydia pneumoniae, Enterobacter cloacae, Klebsiella pneumoniae, Moraxella catarrhalis, Haemophilus influenzae, H. parainfluenzae—**Adult > 18 yr:** 400 mg PO first d as loading dose; then 200 mg/d × 10 d (total, 11 d). *Community-acquired pneumonia from* C. pneumoniae, H. influenzae, H. parainfluenzae, M. catarrhalis, Mycoplasma pneumoniae, S. pneumoniae—**Adult > 18 yr:** 400 mg PO first day as loading dose; then 200 mg/d × 10 d of tx (total, 11 d). ≡ ***Dosage adjustment.*** If CrCl < 50 ml/min, give loading dose of 400 mg PO; then 200 mg PO q 48 h × 9 d of tx (total, six tabs).
stavudine (d4T) • Zerit		
Synthetic thymidine nucleoside analogue; antiviral PRC: C	*Caps:* 15 mg, 20 mg, 30 mg, 40 mg; *Oral sol:* 1 mg/ml	*HIV infect with other antiretrovirals*—**Adult, child weighing ≥ 60 kg:** 40 mg PO q 12 h. **Adult, child weighing 30–60 kg:** 30 mg PO q 12 h. **Child weighing < 30 kg:** 1 mg/kg q 12 h. ≡ ***Dosage adjustment.*** For adult receiving hemodialysis, give 20 mg q 24 h if pt weighs ≥ 60 kg and 15 mg q 24 h if < 60 kg. If adult's CrCl is 26–50 ml/min and pt weighs ≥ 60 kg, give 20 mg q 12 h; if pt weighs < 60 kg, give 15 mg q 12 h. If CrCl is 10–25 ml/min and pt weighs ≥ 60 kg, give 20 mg q 24 h; if pt weighs < 60 kg, give 15 mg q 24 h. Data inadequate for child with renal impairment; consider reducing dose or incr interval.

streptomycin sulfate

Aminoglycoside; antibiotic PRC: D	*Inj:* 400 mg/ml; *Lyophilized cake/pwd for inj:* 200 mg/ ml	*TB*—**Adult:** 15 mg/kg/d (max 1 g/d) IM or 25–30 mg/kg (up to 1.5 g) two to three times/wk × ≥ 1 yr. **Elderly:** Reduced doses/d based on age, renal function, and 8th cranial nerve function. Suggested amt is 10 mg/kg/d (up to 750 mg). **Child:** 20–40 mg/kg/d (up to 1 g) IM or 25–30 mg/kg (up to 1.5 g) two to three times/wk × ≥ 1yr. *Enterococcal endocarditis*—**Adult:** 1 g IM q 12 h × 2 wk; then 500 mg IM q 12 h × 4 wk with PCN. *Tularemia*—**Adult:** 1–2 g/d IM in div doses × 7–14 d or until pt is afebrile × 5–7 d. *Plague*—**Adult:** 2 g/d (30 mg/kg) IM in two div doses × ≥ 10 d. **Child:** 30 mg/kg/d IM in two to three div doses × 10 d. *Brucellosis*—**Adult:** 1 g IM once or twice/d with doxycycline or tetracycline × first wk and once/d × ≥ one more wk. **Child > 8 yr:** 20 mg/kg (up to 1 g) IM in two div doses. *PCN-susceptible streptococcal endocarditis*—**Adult ≥ 60 yr:** 1 g IM twice/d × 1 wk with a PCN. Then 500 mg twice/d × 1 wk. **Adult > 60 yr:** 500 mg twice/d × 2 wk with a PCN. ≡ ***Dosage adjustment.*** Dose and interval based on serum levels (shouldn't peak above 20–25 mcg/ml). If serum levels unavailable, dosage may reflect CrCl. After 1-g loading dose, pt with CrCl 50–80 ml/min should receive 7.5 mg/kg q 24 h. If CrCl 10–50 ml/min, incr interval to q 24–72 h. If CrCl < 10 ml/min, may need q 72–96 h. If pt receives hemodialysis, may give suppl doses 50–75% of loading dose at end of each session. Monitor serum levels and adjust dosage as indicated

Classes	Dosage Forms	Indications & Dosages
sulfacetamide sodium • AK-Sulf, Bleph-10, Cetamide, Isopto Cetamide, Ocusulf-10, Sodium Sulamyd, Storz Sulf, Sulf-10, Sulfair 15, Sulfex ♦, Sulster, Sulten-10		
Sulfonamide; antibiotic PRC: C	*Ophth sol:* 1%, 10%, 15%, 30%; *Ophth oint:* 10%	*Inclusion conjunctivitis, corneal ulcers, trachoma, prophx for ocular infect*—**Adult, child:** 1–2 gtt 10% sol in lower conjunctival sac q 2–3 h during day, less often at night. Or, 1–2 gtt 15% sol in lower conjunctival sac q 1–2 h initially, incr interval as condition responds. Or, 1 gtt 30% sol in lower conjunctival sac q 2 h. Place ½–1″ 10% oint in conjunctival sac qid and hs. Oint may be used at night with gtt during the day. Usual tx lasts 7–10 d.
sulfadiazine		
Sulfonamide; antibiotic PRC: NR	*Tab:* 500 mg	*UTI*— **Adult:** Initially, 2–4 g PO; then 2–4 g/d in three to six div doses. **Child ≥ 2 mo:** Initially, 75 mg/kg or 2 g/m^2 PO; then 150 mg/kg/d PO in four to six div doses. Max, 6 g/d. *Rheumatic fever prophx as alternative to PCN*—**Child weighing > 30 kg:** 1 g/d PO. **Child weighing < 30 kg:** 500 mg/d PO. *Adjunct tx in toxoplasmosis*—**Adult:** 1–1.5 g PO qid × 3–4 wk with pyrimethamine. **Child:** 100–200 mg/kg/d PO in div doses q 6 h × 3–4 wk with pyrimethamine. *Prev of toxoplasmosis relapse in pt with HIV infect*—**Adult, adolescent:** 0.5–1 g PO q 6 h with pyrimethamine and leucovorin. **Infant, child:** 85–120 mg/kg PO in two to four div doses with pyrimethamine and leucovorin. *Nocardiasis*—**Adult:** 4–8 g/d PO in div doses q 6 h × 6 wk. *Asymptomatic meningococcal carrier*—**Adult:** 1 g PO bid × 2 d. **Child 1–12 yr:** 500 mg PO bid × 2 d. **Child 2–12 mo:** 500 mg/d PO × 2 d.

sulfisoxazole, sulfisoxazole acetyl • Gantrisin
sulfisoxazole diolamine • Gantrisin (Ophth Solution)

Sulfonamide; antibiotic PRC: C	*Liq:* 500 mg/5 ml (sulfisoxazole acetyl); *Ophth sol:* 4%; *Tab:* 500 mg	*UTI and systemic infect*—**Adult:** Initially, 2–4 g PO; then 4–8 g/d PO in div doses q 4–6 h. **Child, infant > 2 mo:** Initially, 75 mg/kg PO; then 150 mg/kg/d (or 4 g/m^2) PO in div doses q 4–6 h. Max, 6 g in 24 h. *Conjunctivitis, corneal ulcer, superficial ocular infect, adjunct in systemic tx of trachoma*—**Adult:** 1–2 gtt in lower conjunctival sac of affected eye daily q 1–4 h. ≡ ***Dosage adjustment.*** If CrCl 10–50 ml/min, give dose q 8–12 h. If CrCl < 10 ml/min, give dose q 12–24 h.

tenofovir disoproxil fumarate • Viread

Nucleotide reverse transcriptase inhibitor; antiviral, antiretroviral PRC: B	*Tab:* 300 mg as the fumarate salt (equiv to 245 mg tenofovir disoproxil)	*HIV-1 infect, with other antiretroviral drugs*—**Adult:** 300 mg PO once/d with meal. When given with didanosine, give 2 h before or 1 h after didanosine.

terbinafine hydrochloride • Lamisil, Lamisil AT, Lamisil DermGel

Synthetic allylamine derivative; antifungal PRC: B	**Rx only** *Cream:* 1%; *Gel:* 10 mg/g; *Tab:* 250 mg; **OTC** *Cream:* 1%; *Spray:* 1%	*Interdigital tinea pedis, tinea cruris, or tinea corporis from* Epidermophyton floccosum, Trichophyton mentagrophytes, Trichophyton rubrum—**Adult, child > 12 yr:** For interdigital tinea pedis, apply to affected area and immediate surrounding areas bid until signs and symptoms significantly improve (by d 7 for most pts). For tinea cruris or tinea corporis, apply to affected area and immediate surrounding areas once or twice/d until significant improvement (by d 7 for most pts). Tx should last ≥ 1 wk and ≤ 4 wk. *Onychomycosis of fingernails or toenails from dermatophytes (tinea unguium)*—**Adult, child > 18 yr:** For fingernails, 250 mg/d PO × 6 wk. For toenails, 250 mg/d PO × 12 wk.

Classes	Dosage Forms	Indications & Dosages
terconazole • Terazol 3, Terazol 7		
Triazole derivative; antifungal PRC: C	*Vag cream:* 0.4% in 45-g tube, 0.8% in 20-g tube with applicator; *Vag supp:* 80 mg	*Local tx of vulvovaginal candidiasis*—**Adult:** For 0.4%, 1 full applicator (5 g) intravag once/d hs × 7 d. For 0.8%, 1 full applicator (5 g) intravag once/d hs × 3 d. Or, 1 supp vag hs × 3 d.
tetracycline hydrochloride • Achromycin, Novo-Tetra ♦, Panmycin, Sumycin, Tetracap, Tetracyn, Tetralan, Topicycline		
Tetracycline; antibiotic PRC: D (B, topical)	**Rx only** *Caps:* 100 mg, 250 mg, 500 mg; *Susp:* 125 mg/5 ml; *Tab:* 250 mg, 500 mg; **OTC** *Topical oint:* 3%	*Infect from susceptible organism*—**Adult:** 1–2 g PO in two to four div doses. **Child > 8 yr:** 25–50 mg/kg/d PO in two to four div doses. *Uncomplicated urethral, endocervical, or rectal infect from* Chlamydia trachomatis—**Adult:** 500 mg PO qid × ≥ 7 d. *Brucellosis*—**Adult:** 500 mg PO q 6 h × 3 wk with streptomycin 1 g IM q 12 h during wk 1 and once/d during wk 2. *Gonorrhea in pt sensitive to PCN*—**Adult:** Initially, 1.5 g PO; then 500 mg q 6 h × 4 d. *Syphilis in nonpregnant pt sensitive to PCN*—**Adult:** 500 mg PO qid × 14 d. *Acne*—**Adult, adolescent:** Initially, 500–1,000 mg/d PO, div into four doses; then 125–500 mg/d PO or every other day; apply topical ointment generously to affected areas bid until skin is thoroughly wet. *Lyme disease* ◇—**Adult:** 250–500 mg PO qid × 10–30 d. *Acute transmitted epididymitis (children > 8* ◇*); PID* ◇*; infect with* Helicobacter pylori ◇ *(all use tetracycline as adjunct tx)*—**Adult:** 500 mg PO qid × 10–14 d. *Infect prophx in minor abrasions and tx of superficial infect from susceptible organism*—**Adult, child:** Apply topical oint to infected area one to five times/d.

ticarcillin disodium • Ticar

Alpha-carboxypenicillin; extended-spectrum antibiotic PRC: B	*Inj:* 1 g, 3 g, 6 g; *IV inf:* 3 g	*Serious infect from susceptible organism*—**Adult:** 200–300 mg/kg/d IV, div and given q 4–6 h. **Infant, child > 1 mo weighing < 40 kg:** 200–300 mg/kg/d IV, div and given q 4–6 h. **Neonate weighing > 2 kg:** 225–300 mg/kg/d, div and given q 8 h. **Neonate weighing < 2 kg:** 150–225 mg/kg/d, div and given q 8–12 h. Give prescribed dose IM or by IV inf over 10–20 min. *UTI*—**Adult:** For complicated infect, 150–200 mg/kg/d IV, div and given q 4–6 h. For uncomplicated infect, 1 g IV or IM q 6 h. **Infant, child > 1 mo weighing < 40 kg:** For complicated infect, 150–200 mg/kg/d by IV inf div and given q 4–6 h. For uncomplicated infect, 50–100 mg/kg/d IM or direct IV div and given q 6–8 h. ≡ ***Dosage adjustment.*** For renal impairment, initial loading dose of 3 g IV. If CrCl 30–60 ml/min, give 2 g IV q 4 h. If CrCl 10–30 ml/min, give 2 g IV q 8 h. If CrCl < 10 ml/min, give 2 g IV q 12 h or 1 g IM q 6 h. If CrCl < 10 ml/min and pt also has hepatic impairment, give 2 g IV q 24 h or 1 g IM q 12 h. If pt receives hemodialysis, give 2 g IV q 12 h and 3 g IV after each session. If pt receives peritoneal dialysis, give 3 g IV q 12 h.

ticarcillin disodium/clavulanate potassium • Timentin

Extended-spectrum PCN; beta-lactamase inhibitor, antibiotic PRC: B	*Inj:* 3 g ticarcillin and 100 mg clavulanic acid	*Infect of lower respiratory tract, urinary tract, bones, joints, skin, skin-structure; intraabdominal infect; septicemia from susceptible organism*—**Adult:** 3.1 g (3 g ticarcillin, 100 mg clavulanate potassium) dil in 50–100 ml D_5W, saline sol, or lactated Ringer's inj and given by IV inf over 30 min q 4–6 h. **Child 3 mo to 16 yr weighing < 60 kg:** For mild-to-moderate infect, 200 mg/kg/d (3 g ticarcillin, 100 mg clavulanate potassium) by IV inf in div doses q 6 h. For severe infect, 300 mg/kg/d (3 g ticarcillin, 100 mg clavulanate potassium) IV in div doses q 4 h. *(continued)*

Classes	Dosage Forms	Indications & Dosages
ticarcillin disodium/clavulanate potassium *(continued)*		
		Gyn infect—**Adult weighing ≥ 60 kg:** 200 mg/kg/d indiv doses q 6 h. More severe infect, 300 mg/kg/d in div doses q 4 h. ≡ ***Dosage adjustment.*** In renal impairment, loading dose is 3.1 g (3 g ticarcillin, 100 mg clavulanate). Then, if CrCl 30–60 ml/min, give 2 g IV q 4 h. If CrCl 10–30 ml/min, give 2 g IV q 8 h. If CrCl < 10 ml/min, give 2 g IV q 12 h. If CrCl < 10 ml/min and pt also has hepatic impairment, give 2 g IV q 24 h. If pt receives hemodialysis, give 2 g IV q 12 h with 3.1 g after each session. If pt receives peritoneal dialysis, give 3.1 g IV q 12 h.
tobramycin **tobramycin ophthalmic** • Tobrex **tobramycin sulfate** • Nebcin, Nebcin Add-Vantage ♦, Nebcin Pediatric **tobramycin solution for inhalation** • TOBI		
Aminoglycoside; antibiotic PRC: D	*Inj:* 40 mg/ml, 10 mg/ml (ped), 10 mg/ml (adult); *Neb sol for inhal:* Single-use 5-ml (300-mg) amp; *Ophth sol:* 0.3%; *Ophth oint:* 0.3%	*Serious infect from sensitive* Escherichia coli, Proteus, Klebsiella, Enterobacter, Serratia, Staphylococcus aureus, Pseudomonas, Citrobacter, Providencia—**Adult, child:** 3 mg/kg/d IM or IV, div q 8 h. Up to 5 mg/kg/d IM or IV div q 6–8 h for life-threatening infect. **Neonate < 1 wk:** Up to 4 mg/kg/d IM or IV, div q 12 h. For IV use, dil in 50–100 ml NSS or D_5W for adult, less for child. Infuse over 20–60 min. ≡ ***Dosage adjustment.*** In pt with renal impairment, initial dose unchanged and later doses based on renal function and blood levels; keep peak serum levels at 4–10 mcg/ml and trough levels at 1–2 mcg/ml. After loading dose, reduced doses may be given at 8-h intervals or normal doses may be given at longer than 8-h intervals based on CrCl or creatinine level.

Intrathecal or intraventricular use with IM or IV admin ◇ —**Adult:** 3–8 mg q 18–48 h.

Mgt of cystic fibrosis in pt with Pseudomonas aeruginosa *infect*—**Adult, child > 6 yr:** 1 single-use amp (300 mg) q 12 h × 28 d; then off × 28 d, then on × 28 d as directed.

External ocular infect from susceptible gram-neg bacteria—**Adult, child:** In mild-to-moderate infect, 1–2 gtt in affected eye q 4–6 h. In severe infect, 2 gtt/h in affected eye or place small amt oint in conjunctival sac tid or qid.

tolnaftate • Absorbine Athlete's Foot Cream, Absorbine Footcare, Aftate for Athlete's Foot, Aftate for Jock Itch, Athlete's Foot Powder, Genaspor, Quinsana Plus, Tinactin, Ting

Imidazole derivative; azole antifungal PRC: C	*Aerosol liq:* 1% (36% alcohol); *Aerosol pwd:* 1% (14% alcohol); *Cream:* 1%; *Gel:* 1%; *Pwd:* 1%; *Pump spray liq:* 1% (36% alcohol); *Topical sol:* 1%	*Superficial fungal skin infect; infect from common pathogenic fungi; tinea pedis, tinea cruris, tinea corporis, tinea versicolor*—**Adult, child:** ¼-inch to ½-inch (6-mm to 1.3-cm) ribbon of cream or 2–3 gtt sol to cover area; same amt of cream or sol to cover toes and interdigital webs of one foot; or gel, pwd, or spray to cover affected area. Massage gently into skin bid × 2–6 wk.

triethanolamine polypeptide oleate-condensate • Cerumenex

Oleic acid derivative; ceruminolytic PRC: C	*Otic sol:* 10% in 6-ml and 12-ml bottle with dropper	*Impacted cerumen*—**Adult, child:** Fill ear canal with sol and insert cotton plug. After 15–30 min, flush with warm water using soft rubber bulb ear syringe. Don't leave sol in ear canal > 30 min.

trimethoprim • Primsol, Proloprim, Trimpex

Synthetic folate antagonist; antibiotic PRC: C	*Oral sol:* 50 mg/5 ml; *Tab:* 100 mg, 200 mg	*Uncomplicated UTI from* Escherichia coli, Proteus mirabilis, Klebsiella pnemoniae, Enterobacter sp., *coagluase-neg* Staphylococcus *sp. including* S. saprophyticus *(Primsol)*—**Adult:** 100 mg (10 ml) q 12 h or 200 mg/d (20 ml) × 10 d.

(continued)

Classes	Dosage Forms	Indications & Dosages
trimethoprim *(continued)*		
		Acute otitis media from susceptible Streptococcus pneumoniae *or* Haemophilus influenzae *(Primsol)*—**Child ≥ 6 mo:** 10 mg/kg/d PO in div doses q 12 h × 10 d. *Prophx of chronic, recurrent UTI* ◇ —**Adult:** 100 mg PO hs × 6 wk– 6 mo. *Traveler's diarrhea* ◇ —**Adult:** 200 mg PO bid × 3–5 d. Pneumocystis carinii *pneumonia* ◇ —**Adult:** 5 mg/kg PO tid with dapsone 100 mg/d × 21 d. ≡ ***Dosage adjustment.*** If CrCl 15–30 ml/min, give half usual dose. If CrCl < 15 ml/min, avoid drug.
trovafloxacin mesylate • Trovan **alatrofloxacin mesylate** • Trovan I.V.		
Fluoroquinolone derivative; antibiotic PRC: C	*Tab:* 100 mg, 200 mg; *Inj:* 5 mg/ml, in 40-ml (200 mg) and 60-ml (300 mg) vials	*Gyn, pelvic infect; complicated intra-abdominal including postsurgical infect*—**Adult:** 300 mg/d IV followed by 200 mg/d PO, given once/d × 7–14 d. *Nosocomial pneumonia*—**Adult:** 300 mg IV followed by 200 mg PO, given once/d × 10–14 d. *Community-acquired pneumonia*—**Adult:** 200 mg PO or IV followed by 200 mg PO, given once/d × 7–14 d. *Complicated skin, skin-structure infect, including diabetic foot infect*—**Adult:** 200 mg PO or IV followed by 200 mg PO, given once/d × 10–14 d. ≡ ***Dosage adjustment.*** If pt has mild-to-moderate hepatic disease (cirrhosis), reduce 300 mg IV to 200 mg IV and reduce 200 mg IV or PO to 100 mg IV or PO (no reduction needed for 100 mg PO).

valacyclovir hydrochloride • Valtrex

Synthetic purine nucleoside; antiviral PRC: B	*Capl:* 500 mg, 1,000 mg	*Herpes zoster, immunocompetent pt*—**Adult:** 1 g/d PO tid × 7 d. *Genital herpes initial episode*—**Adult:** 1 g PO bid × 10 d. *Recurrent genital herpes, immunocompetent pt*—**Adult:** 500 mg PO bid × 3 d. *Long-term suppressive therapy, recurrent genital herpes*—**Adult:** 1 g PO once/d. If history of ≤ 9 recurrences/yr, may use 500 mg once/d. ≡ ***Dosage adjustment.*** If CrCl 30–49 ml/min, give 1 g q 12 h for herpes zoster, 500 mg q 12 h for genital herpes. If CrCl 10–29 ml/min, give 1 g q 24 h for herpes zoster, 500 mg q 24 h for genital herpes. If CrCl < 10 ml/min, give 500 mg q 24 h for herpes zoster, 500 mg q 24 h for genital herpes.

valganciclovir hydrochloride • Valcyte

Synthetic nucleoside; antiviral PRC: C	*Tab:* 450 mg	*Active CMV retinitis in pt with AIDS*—**Adult:** 900 mg PO bid with food × 21 d. Maint, 900 mg PO once/d with food. *Inactive CMV retinitis*—**Adult:** 900 mg PO once/d with food. ≡ ***Dosage adjustment.*** For induction, give 450 mg PO bid if CrCl 40–59 ml/min, 450 mg PO once/d if CrCl 25–39 ml/min, or 450 mg PO q 2 d if CrCl 10–24 ml/min. For maint, give 450 mg PO once/d if CrCl 40–59 ml/min, 450 mg PO q 2 d if CrCl 25–39 ml/min, or 450 mg PO twice/wk if CrCl 10–24 ml/min.

vancomycin hydrochloride • Vancocin, Vancoled

Glycopeptide; antibiotic PRC: C	*Pulvules:* 125 mg, 250 mg; *Pwd for inj:* 500-mg, 1-g vials; *Pwd for oral sol:* 1-g, 10-g bottles	*Severe staphylococcal infect when other antibiotics ineffective or contraindicated*—**Adult:** 500 mg IV q 6 h or 1 g q 12 h. **Child:** 40 mg/kg/d IV div q 6 h. **Neonate:** Initially, 15 mg/kg Then, 10 mg/kg IV q 12 h for first wk after birth. Then, q 8 h to age 1 mo. *Antibiotic-related pseudomembranous and staphylococcal enterocolitis*—**Adult:** 125–500 mg PO q 6 h × 7–10 d. **Child:** 40 mg/kg/d *(continued)*

Classes	Dosage Forms	Indications & Dosages
vancomycin hydrochloride *(continued)*		
		PO div q 6–8 h × 7–10 d. Max 2 g/d in child. *Endocarditis prophyx for dental, GI, biliary, GU instrument procedures; surg prophx in pt allergic to PCN*—**Adult:** 1 g IV slowly over 1–2 h with inf complete ≤ 30 min after procedure starts. **Child:** 20 mg/kg IV slowly over 1–2 h with inf complete ≤ 30 min after procedure starts. ≡ ***Dosage adjustment.*** Dosage adjusted based on amt of renal impairment, severity of infect, susceptibility of organism, drug levels. Initial dose usually 15 mg/kg, then adjusted prn. Some recommend 1 g q 12 h if creatinine < 1.5 mg/dl;1 g q 3–6 d if creatinine 1.5–5 mg/dl; 1 g q 10–14 d if creatinine > 5 mg/dl.
vidarabine (adenine arabinoside) • Vira-A		
Purine nucleoside; antiviral PRC: C	*Ophth oint:* 3% in 3.5-g tube (equiv to 2.8% vidarabine)	*Acute keratoconjunctivitis, recurrent epithelial keratitis from HSV types 1, 2*—**Adult, child**: ¼-inch (1.3 cm) oint in lower conjunctival sac five times/d at 3-h intervals.
zalcitabine (dideoxycytidine, ddC) • Hivid		
Nucleoside analogue; antiretroviral PRC: C	*Tab (film-coated):* 0.375 mg, 0.75 mg	*HIV infect, with other retroviral agents*—**Adult, child ≥ 13 yr:** 0.75 mg PO q 8 h. ≡ ***Dosage adjustment.*** If CrCl 10–40 ml/min, give 0.75 mg PO q 12 h. If CrCl < 10 ml/min, give 0.75 mg PO q 24 h.
zanamivir • Relenza		
Neuraminidase inhibitor; antiviral PRC: C	*Pwd for inhal:* 5 mg per blister pack	*Uncomplicated acute illness from influenza A or B virus in pt symptomatic ≤ 2 d*—**Adult, child ≥ 7 yr:** 2 inhal q 12 h × 5 d.

zidovudine (AZT) • Retrovir

Thymidine analogue; antiviral
PRC: C

Caps: 100 mg; *Inj:* 10 mg/ml; *Syrup:* 50 mg/5 ml; *Tab:* 300 mg

HIV infect—**Adult:** 600 mg/d PO in div doses with other antiretroviral drugs. **Child 6 wk–12 yr:** 160 mg/m^2 PO q 8 h (480 mg/m^2/d to max of 200 mg q 8 h) with other antiretroviral drugs.

Prev of maternal-fetal HIV transmission—**Pregnant woman > 14 wk gestation:** 100 mg PO five times/d until labor starts. Then, 2 mg/kg IV over 1 h followed by cont IV inf of 1 mg/kg/h until umbilical cord clamped. **Neonate:** 2 mg/kg PO q 6 h starting ≤ 12 h after birth and cont until 6 wk old. Or, 1.5 mg/kg via IV inf over 30 min q 6 h.

≡ ***Dosage adjustment.*** Drug may need interruption if pt has significant anemia (hemoglobin < 7.5 g/dl or reduction > 25% of baseline) or neutropenia (granulocyte count < 750 cells/mm^3 or reduction > 50% of baseline) until evidence of marrow recovery. If pt receives hemodialysis or peritoneal dialysis, give 100 mg PO q 6–8 h. If pt has mild-to-moderate hepatic dysfunction or cirrhosis, dose may need reduction.

Therapeutic monitoring guidelines

The table below lists laboratory tests, therapeutic ranges, and guidelines for monitoring patient response to common anti-infectives.

Drug	Laboratory test monitored	Therapeutic ranges of test
aminoglycosides (amikacin, gentamicin, tobramycin)	Serum amikacin peak trough Serum gentamicin/ tobramycin peak trough Serum creatinine	20–30 mcg/ml 5–10 mcg/ml 4–10 mcg/ml 1–2 mcg/ml 0.6–1.3 mg/dl
amphotericin B	Serum creatinine BUN Serum electrolytes (especially potassium and magnesium) Liver function tests CBC with differential and platelets	0.6–1.3 mg/dl 7–18 mg/dl Potassium: 3.5–5 mEq/L Magnesium: 1.7–2.1 mEq/L Sodium: 135–145 mEq/L Chloride: 98–106 mEq/L * *****
antibiotics	WBC with differential cultures and sensitivities	*****
antituberculotics	Liver function tests Uric acid	* 3–8 mg/dl

***** For those areas marked with asterisks, the following values can be used:

Hgb: Women: 12–16 g/dl
Men: 14–18 g/dl
Hct: Women: 37%–48%
Men: 42%–52%
RBCs: 4–5.5 x 10^6/mm^3
WBCs: 5–10 x 10^3/mm^3

Differential: Neutrophils: 45%–74%
Bands: 0%–4%
Lymphocytes: 16%–45%
Monocytes: 4%–0%
Eosinophils: 0%–7%
Basophils: 0%–2%

Monitoring guidelines

Wait until giving third dose to check drug levels. Obtain blood for peak level 30 min after IV inf or 60 min after IM admin. For trough levels, draw blood just before next dose. Adjust dosage accordingly. Recheck after three doses. Monitor serum creatinine, BUN, and urine output for decreasing renal function. Monitor WBC wkly during tx. Monitor culture and sensitivity results to determine causative agent and appropriate tx.

Monitor serum creatinine, BUN, and urine output for signs of decreasing renal function. Monitor electrolytes, especially potassium and magnesium. Monitor pt for signs of hypokalemia (cramping, muscle weakness, ECG changes). Blood counts, temperature, and liver function tests should also be monitored regularly during tx.

Specimen cultures and sensitivities will determine the cause of the infect and the appropriate tx. Monitor WBC with differential wkly during tx. Any change in liver or kidney function may require a dosage adjustment.

Obtain liver function tests at baseline and q 1–3 mo during tx. Consult pharmacist when adding or removing drugs because antituberculotics can affect other drugs' levels and potency.

(continued)

* For those areas marked with one asterisk, the following values can be used:

ALT: 7–56 U/L
AST: 5–40 U/L
Alkaline phosphatase: 17–142 U/L
LDH: 60–220 U/L
GGT: < 40 U/L
Total bilirubin: 0.2–1 mg/dl

Drug	Laboratory test monitored	Therapeutic ranges of test
antivirals	Serum creatinine	0.6–1.3 mg/dl
	CBC and platelets	*****
protease inhibitors	HIV RNA levels	
	CD4+ T-cell count	
	Total cholesterol	< 200 mg/dl
	Triglycerides	40–60 mg/dl
	Serum glucose	65–110 mg/dl
vancomycin	Serum vancomycin	5–10 mcg/ml (trough)
	Serum creatinine	0.6–1.3 mg/dl

***** For those areas marked with asterisks, the following values can be used:

Hgb: Women: 12–16 g/dl
Men: 14–18 g/dl
Hct: Women: 37%–48%
Men: 42%–52%
RBCs: 4–5.5 x 10^6/mm^3
WBCs: 5–10 x 10^3/mm^3

Differential: Neutrophils: 45%–74%
Bands: 0%–4%
Lymphocytes: 16%–45%
Monocytes: 4%–10%
Eosinophils: 0%–7%
Basophils: 0%–2%

Monitoring guidelines

Monitor serum creatinine, BUN, and urine output during tx. Blood counts and liver function tests should also be monitored during tx.

Obtain HIV RNA level and CD4+ T-cell count at baseline, 2–8 wk after tx starts to eval effectiveness, and q 3–4 mo to eval durability of response. Protease inhibitors can cause hyperglyceima and dyslipidemia, which includes elevated cholesterol and triglyceride levels. Consult with pharmacist before adding or removing any drugs because protease inhibitors have complex metabolism and may have drug-drug interactions.

Serum vancomycin level may be checked with third dose given (at the earliest). Trough levels should be drawn immed before giving next dose. Renal function can be used to adjust dosing and intervals. Monitor culture and sensitivity results to determine causative agent. Monitor WBC and differential wkly during tx.

* For those areas marked with one asterisk, the following values can be used:

ALT: 7–56 U/L
AST: 5–40 U/L
Alkaline phosphatase: 17–142 U/L
LDH: 60–220 U/L
GGT: < 40 U/L
Total bilirubin: 0.2–1 mg/dl

Comparing penicillins

The table below lists selected penicillins and their dosage requirements. It also indicates whether or not they are penicillinase-resistant.

Drug	Route	Adult dose	Frequency	Penicillinase-resistant
amoxicillin	PO	250–500 mg	q 8 h	No
amoxicillin/ clavulanate potassium	PO	250 mg 500 mg 875 mg	q 8 h q 8–12 h q 12 h	Yes
ampicillin	IM, IV	2–14 g daily	divided doses given q 4–6 h	No
	PO	250–500 mg	q 6 h	
ampicillin sodium/ sulbactam sodium	IM, IV	1.5–3 g	q 6–8 h	Yes
carbenicillin	PO	382–764 mg	q 6 h	No
cloxacillin	PO	250 mg–1 g	q 6 h	Yes
dicloxacillin	PO	125–500 mg	q 6 h	Yes
mezlocillin	IM, IV	3–4 g	q 4–6 h	No
nafcillin	IM, IV PO	250 mg–2 g 500 mg–1 g	q 4–6 h q 6 h	Yes
oxacillin	IM, IV PO	250 mg–2 g 500 mg–1 g	q 4–6 h q 6 h	Yes
penicillin G benzathine	IM	1.2–2.4 million units	single dose	No
penicillin G potassium	IM, IV	200,000–4 million units	q 4 h	No

Drug	Route	Adult dose	Frequency	Penicillinase-resistant
penicillin G procaine	IM	600,000–2.4 million units	once/d	No
penicillin G sodium	IM, IV	200,000–4 million units	q 4 h	No
penicillin V potassium	PO	250–500 mg	q 6–8 h	No
piperacillin	IM, IV	3–4 g	q 4–6 h	No
piperacillin sodium/ tazobactam sodium	IV	3.375 g 4.5 g	q 6 h q 8 h	Yes
ticarcillin disodium	IM, IV	3–4 g	q 4–6 h	No
ticarcillin/ clavulanate potassium	IV	3.1 g	q 4–6 h	Yes

Comparing cephalosporins

The table below lists selected cephalosporins and their elimination half-life, sodium content, and CSF penetration.

Drug and route	Elimination half-life (h)		Sodium (mEq/g)	CSF penetration
	Normal renal function	End-stage renal disease		
cefaclor PO	0.5–1	2–3	Unknown	No
cefadroxil PO	1–2	20–25	Unknown	No
cefamandole IM, IV	0.5–2	12–18	Unknown	No
cefazolin IM, IV	1.2–2.2	3–7	2–2.1	No
cefdinir PO	1.5	16	Unknown	Unknown
cefditoren PO	1.6	Unknown	Unknown	Unknown
cefepime IM, IV	2	17–21	Unknown	Yes
cefixime PO	3–4	11.5	Unknown	Unknown
cefmetazole IV	1.2	Unknown	2	Unknown
cefonicid IM, IV	3.5–5.8	11	3.7	No
cefoperazone IM, IV	1.5–2.5	1.3–2.9	1.5	Sometimes
cefotaxime IM, IV	1–1.5	3–11	2.2	Yes

Drug and route	Elimination half-life (h)		Sodium (mEq/g)	CSF penetration
	Normal renal function	End-stage renal disease		
cefotetan IM, IV	2.8–4.6	13–35	3.5	No
cefoxitin IV	0.5–1	6.5–21.5	2.3	No
cefpodoxime PO	2–3	9.8	Unknown	Unknown
cefprozil PO	1–1.5	5.2–5.9	Unknown	Unknown
ceftazidime IM, IV	1.5–2	14–30	2.3	Yes
ceftibuten PO	2.4	13.4–22.3	Unknown	Unknown
ceftizoxime IM, IV	1.5–2	25–30	2.6	Yes
ceftriaxone IM, IV	5.5–11	15.7	3.6	Yes
cefuroxime PO, IM, IV	1–2	15–22	2.4	Yes (IM, IV)
cephalexin PO	0.5–1	19–22	Unknown	No
cephapirin IM, IV	0.5–1	2–4	2.4	No
cephradine PO, IM, IV	0.5–2	8–15	6	No

Aminoglycosides: Renal function and half-life

Aminoglycosides, which are excreted by the kidneys, have significantly prolonged half-lives in patients with end-stage renal disease. Knowing this can help you assess the patient's potential for drug accumulation and toxicity. Nephrotoxicity, a major hazard of therapy with aminoglycosides, is linked to serum levels that exceed the therapeutic levels listed below. Therefore, monitoring peak and trough levels is essential for safe use of these drugs.

	Half-life (h)		Therapeutic levels (mcg/ml)	
Drug and route	**Normal renal function**	**End-stage renal disease**	**Peak**	**Trough**
amikacin IM, IV	2–3	24–60	16–32	< 10
gentamicin IM, IV, topical	2	24–60	4–10	< 2
kanamycin IM, IV, topical	2–3	24–60	15–40	< 10
neomycin PO, topical	2–3	12–24	Not applicable	Not applicable
netilmicin IM, IV	2–2.7	< 40	6–10	< 2
streptomycin IM, IV	2.5	100	20–30	Not applicable
tobramycin IM, IV, topical	2–2.5	24–60	4–10	< 2

Dialyzable anti-infectives

The amount of a drug removed by dialysis differs among patients and depends on several factors, including the patient's condition, the drug's properties, length of dialysis and dialysate used, rate of blood flow or dwell time, and purpose of dialysis. This table indicates the effect of hemodialysis on selected drugs.

Drug	Level reduced by hemodialysis
acyclovir	Yes
amikacin	Yes
amoxicillin	Yes
amoxicillin and clavulanate potassium	Yes
amphotericin B	No
ampicillin	Yes
ampicillin and sulbactam sodium	Yes
aztreonam	Yes
carbenicillin	Yes
cefaclor	Yes
cefadroxil	Yes
cefamandole	Yes
cefazolin	Yes
cefepime	Yes
cefonicid	Yes (by 20%)
cefoperazone	Yes
cefotaxime	Yes
cefotetan	Yes (by 20%)
cefoxitin	Yes
ceftazidime	Yes
ceftizoxime	Yes
ceftriaxone	No
cefuroxime	Yes
cephalexin	Yes
cephalothin	Yes
cephapirin	Yes
chloroquine	No
ciprofloxacin	Yes (by 20%)
clindamycin	No
cloxacillin	No
co-trimoxazole	Yes
dicloxacillin	No
doxycycline	No
erythromycin	Yes (by 20%)
ethambutol	Yes (by 20%)
fluconazole	Yes
flucytosine	Yes
ganciclovir	Yes
gentamicin	Yes
imipenem and cilastatin sodium	Yes
isoniazid	Yes
kanamycin	Yes

(continued)

Drug	Level reduced by hemodialysis
ketoconazole	No
levofloxacin	No
loracarbef	Yes
metronidazole	Yes
mezlocillin	Yes
miconazole	No
minocycline	No
nafcillin	No
nelfinavir	No
netilmicin	Yes
norfloxacin	No
ofloxacin	Yes
penicillin G	Yes
pentamidine	No
piperacillin	Yes
quinidine	Yes
rifampin	No
stavudine	Yes
streptomycin	Yes
sulbactam	Yes
ticarcillin	Yes
tobramycin	Yes
trimethoprim	Yes
valacyclovir	Yes
vancomycin	No

Gram-positive and gram-negative aerobes

Gram-positive (+) aerobes

Gram-positive bacteria have simple cell walls. These cells are impermeable to organic solvents and retain the purple dye applied during the Gram staining procedure. Gram-positive aerobes commonly appear where the body is exposed to a lot of oxygen, such as the skin and the surfaces of upper respiratory tract structures. Below is a list of gram-positive aerobes.

- Bacillus anthracis
- Campylobacter jejuni
- Clostridium difficile
- Clostridium perfringens
- Enterococcus faecalis
- Enterococcus faecium
- Listeria monocytogenes
- Nocardia asteroids
- Staphylococcus aureus
- Staphylococcus saprophyticus
- Streptococcus pneumoniae
- Streptococcus pyogenes (group A)
- Streptococcus (anaerobic sp.)
- Streptococcus (viridans group)

Gram-negative (-) aerobes

Gram-negative bacteria have complex, lipid-rich cell walls. Because they are permeable to organic solvents, cells decolorize and counterstain red during the Gram staining procedure. In general, gram-negative aerobes are commonly pathogenic in the GI, GU, and lower respiratory tract, although they may cause disease in any body system. Below is a list of gram-negative aerobes.

- Acinetobacter
- Bacteroides fragilis
- Chlamydia pneumoniae
- Chlamydia psittaci
- Chlamydia trachomatis
- Citrobacter fruendii
- Enterobacter sp.
- Escherichia coli
- Haemophilus influenzae
- Klebsiella pneumoniae (UTI)
- Klebsiella pneumoniae (pneumonia)
- Legionella pneumophila
- Moraxella catarrhalis
- Neisseria gonorrhoeae
- Proteus mirabilis
- Proteus vulgaris
- Pseudomonas aeruginosa
- Serratia marcescens
- Shigella sp.
- Vibrio cholerae

Comparing types of pneumonia

Type	Signs and symptoms
Influenza	▪ Cough (initially nonproductive; later, purulent sputum), marked cyanosis, dyspnea, high fever, chills, substernal pain and discomfort, moist crackles, frontal headache, and myalgia
Adenovirus	▪ Sore throat, fever, cough, chills, malaise, small amounts of mucoid sputum, retrosternal chest pain, anorexia, rhinitis, adenopathy, scattered crackles, and rhonchi
Respiratory syncytial virus	▪ Listlessness, irritability, tachypnea with retraction of intercostal muscles, wheezing, slight sputum production, fine moist crackles, fever, severe malaise, and, possibly, cough or croup
Measles (rubeola)	▪ Fever, dyspnea, cough, small amounts of sputum, coryza, rash, and cervical adenopathy
Chickenpox (varicella)	▪ Cough, dyspnea, cyanosis, tachypnea, pleuritic chest pain, hemoptysis, and rhonchi 1 to 6 days after onset of rash
Cytomegalovirus	▪ Fever, cough, shaking chills, dyspnea, cyanosis, weakness, and diffuse crackles ▪ Occurs in neonates as devastating multisystemic infection; in adults resembles mononucleosis; in immunocompromised patients, varies from clinically inapparent to devastating infection

Diagnosis	Treatment
• *Chest X-ray:* diffuse bilateral bronchopneumonia from hilus • *WBC count:* normal to slightly elevated; lymphocytic predominance • *Sputum smears:* no specific organisms	• *Supportive:* for respiratory failure, endotracheal intubation and ventilator assistance; for fever, hypothermia blanket or antipyretics; for influenza A, amantadine or rimantadine
• *Chest X-ray:* patchy distribution of pneumonia, more severe than indicated by physical examination • *WBC count:* normal to slightly elevated	• Symptomatic treatment only • Mortality low, usually clears with no residual effects
• *Chest X-ray:* patchy bilateral consolidation • *WBC count:* normal to slightly elevated	• *Supportive:* humidified air, oxygen, antimicrobials often given until viral etiology confirmed, aerosolized ribavirin • Complete recovery in 1 to 3 weeks
• *Chest X-ray:* reticular infiltrates, sometimes with hilar lymph node enlargement • *Lung tissue specimen:* characteristic giant cells	• *Supportive:* bed rest, adequate hydration, antimicrobials; assisted ventilation, if necessary
• *Chest X-ray:* shows more extensive pneumonia than indicated by physical examination, and bilateral, patchy, diffuse, nodular infiltrates • *Sputum analysis:* predominant mononuclear cells and characteristic intranuclear inclusion bodies with skin rash confirm diagnosis	• *Supportive:* adequate hydration, oxygen therapy in critically ill patients • Therapy with IV acyclovir
• *Chest X-ray:* in early stages, variable patchy infiltrates; later, bilateral, nodular, and more predominant in lower lobes • Difficult to distinguish from other nonbacterial pneumonias • *Percutaneous aspiration of lung tissue, transbronchial biopsy or open lung biopsy:* microscopic examination shows intranuclear and cytoplasmic inclusions; virus can be cultured from lung tissue	• Generally, benign and self-limiting in mononucleosis-like form • *Supportive:* adequate hydration and nutrition, oxygen therapy, bed rest • In immunosuppressed patients, disease more severe and possibly fatal, ganciclovir or foscarnet treatment warranted

(continued)

Type	**Signs and symptoms**
Streptococcus (Diplococcus pneumoniae)	• Sudden onset of a single, shaking chill, and sustained temperature of 102° to 104° F (38.9° to 40° C), often preceded by upper respiratory tract infection
Klebsiella	• Fever and recurrent chills; cough producing rusty, bloody, viscous sputum (currant jelly); cyanosis of lips and nail beds due to hypoxemia; shallow, grunting respirations • Common in patients with chronic alcoholism, pulmonary disease, diabetes, and those at risk for aspiration
Staphylococcus	• Temperature of 102° to 104° F (38.9° to 40° C), recurrent shaking chills, bloody sputum, dyspnea, tachypnea, and hypoxemia • Should be suspected with viral illness, such as influenza or measles, and in patients with cystic fibrosis
Pneumocystis carinii	• Occurs in immunocompromised patients • Dyspnea and nonproductive cough • Anorexia, weight loss, and fatigue • Low-grade fever
Aspiration	• Noncardiogenic pulmonary edema may follow damage to respiratory epithelium from contact with stomach acid • Crackles, dyspnea, cyanosis, hypotension, and tachycardia • Possibly subacute pneumonia with cavity formation, or lung abscess if foreign body is present

Diagnosis	Treatment
▪ *Chest X-ray:* areas of consolidation, often lobar ▪ *WBC count:* elevated ▪ *Sputum culture:* may show gram-positive *S. pneumoniae;* this organism not always recovered	▪ *Antimicrobial therapy:* macrolide for 7 to 10 days; begun after obtaining culture specimen but without waiting for results
▪ *Chest X-ray:* typically, but not always, consolidation in the upper lobe that causes bulging of fissures ▪ *WBC count:* elevated ▪ *Sputum culture and Gram stain:* may show gram-negative cocci *(Klebsiella)*	▪ *Antimicrobial therapy:* an aminoglycoside and a cephalosporin
▪ *Chest X-ray:* multiple abscesses and infiltrates; high incidence of empyema ▪ *WBC count:* elevated ▪ *Sputum culture and Gram stain:* may show gram-positive staphylococci	▪ *Antimicrobial therapy:* nafcillin or oxacillin for 14 days if staphylococci are penicillinase producing ▪ *Supportive:* Chest tube drainage of empyema
▪ *Fiber-optic bronchoscopy:* obtains specimens for histologic studies ▪ *Chest X-ray:* nonspecific infiltrates, nodular lesions, or spontaneous pneumothorax	▪ *Antimicrobial therapy:* co-trimoxazole or pentamidine by IV or inhalation ▪ *Supportive:* oxygen, improved nutrition, mechanical ventilation
▪ *Chest X-ray:* locates areas of infiltrates, which suggest diagnosis	▪ *Antimicrobial therapy:* penicillin G or clindamycin ▪ *Supportive:* oxygen therapy, suctioning, coughing, deep breathing, adequate hydration

Comparing streptococcal infections

Infections and characteristics	Signs and symptoms
Streptococcus pyogenes (Group A streptococcus)	
Streptococcal pharyngitis (strep throat) ▪ Accounts for 95% of all cases of bacterial pharyngitis ▪ Most common in children ages 5 to 10 from October to April ▪ Spread by direct person-to-person contact via droplets of saliva or nasal secretions ▪ Usually colonizes throats of patients with no symptoms; up to 20% of school children possible carriers; pets also possible carriers	▪ After 1- to 5-day incubation period: temperature of 101° to 104° F (38.3° to 40° C), sore throat with severe pain on swallowing, beefy red pharynx, tonsillar exudate, edematous tonsils and uvula, swollen glands along the jaw line, generalized malaise and weakness, headaches, occasional abdominal discomfort ▪ In up to 40% of small children, symptoms too mild for diagnosis ▪ Fever abating in 3 to 5 days; nearly all symptoms subsiding within a week
Scarlet fever (scarlatina) ▪ Usually follows streptococcal pharyngitis; may follow wound infections or puerperal sepsis ▪ Caused by streptococcal strain that releases an erythrogenic toxin ▪ Most common in children ages 2 to 10 ▪ Spread by inhalation or direct contact	▪ Streptococcal sore throat, fever, strawberry tongue, fine erythematous rash that blanches on pressure and resembles sunburn with goosebumps ▪ Rash usually appearing first on upper chest, then spreading to neck, abdomen, legs, and arms, sparing soles and palms; lushed cheeks; pallor around mouth ▪ Skin shedding during convalescence

Diagnosis	Complications	Treatment and special considerations
• Clinically indistinguishable from viral pharyngitis • Throat culture showing group A beta-hemolytic streptococci (carriers have positive throat culture) • Elevated WBC count • A four-fold rise in streptozyme titers during convalescence	• Most frequently, acute otitis media or acute sinusitis • Rarely, bacteremic spread may cause arthritis, endocarditis, meningitis, osteomyelitis, or liver abscess • Poststreptococcal sequelae: acute rheumatic fever or acute glomerulonephritis • Reye's syndrome	• Penicillin or erythromycin, analgesics, and antipyretics • Bed rest and isolation from other children for 24 hours after antibiotic therapy begins • Full compliance with antibiotic treatment with no skipped doses, even if symptoms subside, to avoid abscess, glomerulonephritis, and rheumatic fever • Proper disposal of soiled tissues
• Characteristic rash and strawberry tongue • Culture and Gram stain showing *S. pyogenes* from nasopharynx • Granulocytosis	• Rarely, high fever, arthritis, jaundice, pneumonia, pericarditis, and peritonsillar abscess	• Penicillin or erythromycin • Isolation for first 24 hours • Careful disposal of purulent discharge • Prompt and complete antibiotic treatment

(continued)

Infections and characteristics	Signs and symptoms
Streptococcus pyogenes (Group A streptococcus) *(continued)*	
Erysipelas ▪ Occurs primarily in infants and adults over age 30 ▪ Usually follows strep throat ▪ Exact mode of spread to skin unknown	▪ Sudden onset, with reddened, swollen, raised lesions that sting and itch (skin resembles orange peel), usually on face and scalp, bordered by areas that often contain easily ruptured blebs filled with yellow-tinged fluid (Lesions on the trunk, arms, or legs usually affect incision or wound sites.) ▪ Other symptoms: vomiting, fever, headache, cervical lymphadenopathy, sore throat
Impetigo (streptococcal pyoderma) ▪ Common in poor children ages 2 to 5 in hot, humid weather; high rate of familial spread ▪ Predisposing factors: close contact in schools, overcrowded living quarters, poor skin hygiene, minor skin trauma ▪ May spread by direct contact, environmental contamination, or arthropod vector	▪ Small macules that rapidly develop into vesicles, then become pustular and encrusted, causing pain, surrounding erythema, regional adenitis, cellulitis, and itching; infection spread by scratching ▪ Lesions that commonly affect the face, heal slowly, and leave depigmented areas
Streptococcal gangrene (necrotizing fasciitis) ▪ More common in elderly patients with arteriosclerotic vascular disease or diabetes ▪ Predisposing factors: surgery, wounds, skin ulcers, diabetes, peripheral vascular disease ▪ Spread by direct contact	▪ Mimics gas gangrene; within 72 hours of onset, red-streaked, painful skin lesions with dusky red surrounding tissue; then, development and rupture of bullae with yellow or reddish black fluid ▪ Other signs and symptoms: fever, tachycardia, lethargy, prostration, disorientation, hypotension, jaundice, hypovolemia, severe pain followed by anesthesia (due to nerve destruction)

Diagnosis	Complications	Treatment and special considerations
• Typical reddened lesions • Culture taken from edge of lesions showing group A beta-hemolytic streptococci • Throat culture almost always positive for group A beta-hemolytic streptococci	• Untreated lesions on trunk, arms, or legs possibly involving large body areas and leading to death	• Penicillin or erythromycin IV or PO • Cold packs, analgesics (aspirin and codeine for local discomfort), topical anesthetics • Prevention: prompt treatment of streptococcal infections, and drainage and secretion precautions
• Characteristic lesions with honey-colored crust • Culture and Gram stain of swabbed lesions showing *S. pyogenes*	• Septicemia (rare) • Ecthyma, a form of impetigo with deep ulcers	• Penicillin IV or PO, or erythromycin, or antibiotic ointments • Frequent washing of lesions with antiseptics, followed by thorough drying • Isolation of patient with draining wounds • Good hygiene and proper wound care
• Culture and Gram stain usually showing *S. pyogenes* from early bullous lesions and commonly from blood	• Extensive necrotic sloughing • Bacteremia, metastatic abscesses, and death • Thrombophlebitis, when legs are involved	• Immediate, wide, deep surgery of all necrotic tissues • High-dose penicillin IV • Good preoperative skin preparation, aseptic surgical and suturing technique

(continued)

Infections and characteristics	Signs and symptoms
Streptococcus agalactiae (Group B streptococcus)	
Neonatal streptococcal infection ▪ Incidence of early-onset infection (age 5 days or less): 2/1,000 live births ▪ Incidence of late-onset infection (age 7 days to 3 months): 1/1,000 live births ▪ Predisposing factors: maternal genital tract colonization, membrane rupture over 24 hours before delivery, vaginal delivery, crowded nursery	▪ Early onset: bacteremia, pneumonia, and meningitis; mortality from 14% for infants over 1,500 g at birth to 61% for infants under 1,500 g at birth ▪ Late onset: bacteremia with meningitis, fever, and bone and joint involvement; mortality 15% to 20% ▪ Other signs and symptoms, such as skin lesions, depending on site
Adult group B streptococcal infection ▪ Most adult infections occur in postpartum women, usually in the form of endometritis or wound infection following cesarean section ▪ Incidence of group B streptococcal endometritis: 1.3/1,000 live births	▪ Fever, malaise, uterine tenderness ▪ Change in lochia
Streptococcus pneumoniae (Group D streptococcus)	
Pneumococcal pneumonia ▪ Accounts for 70% of all cases of bacterial pneumonia ▪ More common in men, elderly people, Blacks, and Native Americans, in winter and early spring ▪ Spread by air and contact with infective secretions ▪ Predisposing factors: trauma, viral infection, underlying pulmonary disease, overcrowded living quarters, chronic diseases, immunodeficiency ▪ Among the 10 leading causes of death in the United States	▪ Sudden onset with severe shaking chills, temperature of 102° to 105° F (38.9° to 40.6° C), bacteremia, cough (with thick, scanty, blood-tinged sputum) accompanied by pleuritic pain ▪ Malaise, weakness, and prostration common ▪ Tachypnea, anorexia, nausea, and vomiting less common ▪ Severity of pneumonia usually due to patient's cellular defenses, not bacterial virulence

Diagnosis	Complications	Treatment and special considerations
▪ Isolation of group B streptococcus from blood, CSF, or skin ▪ Chest X-ray showing massive infiltrate similar to that of respiratory distress syndrome or pneumonia	▪ Overwhelming pneumonia, sepsis, and death	▪ Penicillin or ampicillin and an aminoglycoside IV ▪ Patient isolation if open draining lesion is present ▪ Careful hand washing; drainage and secretion precautions, if draining lesion is present ▪ Vaccine in development
▪ Isolation of group B streptococcus from blood or infection site	▪ Bacteremia followed by meningitis or endocarditis	▪ Ampicillin or penicillin IV ▪ Observe for symptoms of infection after delivery ▪ Drainage and secretion precautions
▪ Gram stain of sputum showing gram-positive diplococci; culture showing *S. pneumoniae* ▪ Chest X-ray showing lobular consolidation in adults; bronchopneumonia in children and in elderly patients ▪ Elevated WBC count ▪ Blood cultures often positive for *S. pneumoniae*	▪ Pleural effusion occurs in 25% of patients ▪ Pericarditis (rare) ▪ Lung abscess (rare) ▪ Bacteremia followed by meningitis or endocarditis ▪ Disseminated intravascular coagulation ▪ Death possible if bacteremia is present	▪ Penicillin or erythromycin IV or IM ▪ Respiratory monitoring and support as needed; recording of sputum color and amount ▪ Fluids to prevent dehydration ▪ Avoidance of sedatives and narcotics to preserve cough reflex ▪ Careful disposal of all purulent drainage (respiratory isolation unnecessary)

(continued)

Infections and characteristics	Signs and symptoms
Streptococcus pnuemoniae (Group D streptococcus) *(continued)*	
Pneumococcal pneumonia *(continued)*	
Otitis media	
▪ Occurring at least once in about 76% to 95% of all children, with *S. pneumoniae* causing half of these cases	▪ Ear pain, ear drainage, hearing loss, fever, lethargy, irritability ▪ Other possible symptoms include vertigo, nystagmus, tinnitus
Meningitis	
▪ Can follow bacteremic pneumonia, mastoiditis, sinusitis, skull fracture, or endocarditis ▪ Mortality (30% to 60%) highest in infants and in elderly patients	▪ Fever, headache, nuchal rigidity, vomiting, photophobia, lethargy, coma, wide pulse pressure, bradycardia
Endocarditis	
▪ Group D streptococcus (enterococcus) causes 10% to 20% of all bacterial endocarditis ▪ Most common in elderly patients and in those who abuse IV substances ▪ Often follows bacteremia from an obvious source, such as a wound infection, urinary tract infection, or IV insertion site infection ▪ Most cases subacute	▪ Weakness, fatigue, weight loss, fever, night sweats, anorexia, arthralgia, splenomegaly, new systolic murmur

Diagnosis	Complications	Treatment and special considerations
		▪ For high-risk patients, vaccine and avoidance of infected persons
▪ Fluid in middle ear ▪ Isolation of *S. pneumoniae* from aspirated fluid if necessary	▪ Possible hearing loss from recurrent attacks	▪ Amoxicillin or ampicillin and analgesics ▪ Patient to report lack of response to therapy after 72 hours
▪ Isolation of *S. pneumoniae* from CSF or blood culture ▪ Increased CSF cell count and protein level; decreased CSF glucose level ▪ Computed tomography scan of head ▪ EEG	▪ Persistent hearing deficits, seizures, hemiparesis, or other nerve deficits ▪ Encephalitis	▪ Penicillin IV or chloramphenicol ▪ Close monitoring for neurologic changes and symptoms of septic shock, such as acidosis and tissue hypoxia
▪ Anemia, increased erythrocyte sedimentation rate and serum immunoglobulin level, and positive blood culture for group D streptococcus ▪ ECG showing vegetation on valves	▪ Embolization ▪ Pulmonary infarction ▪ Osteomyelitis	▪ Penicillin for *Streptococcus bovis* (nonenterococcal group D streptococcus) ▪ Penicillin or ampicillin and an aminoglycoside for enterococcal group D streptococcus

Facts about anthrax

Bacillus anthracis, the etiologic agent of anthrax, is a large, gram-positive, non-motile, spore-forming bacterial rod. The three virulence factors of *B. anthracis* are edema toxin, lethal toxin, and a capsular antigen. Anthrax has three major clinical forms: cutaneous, inhalation, and gastrointestinal. If left untreated, anthrax in all forms can lead to septicemia and death. Early diagnosis and treatment of all forms is important for recovery. Any suspected isolate of *Bacillus anthracis* or any suspected case of anthrax must be immediately reported to the local or state public health department. The lists below gives characterictics of the three types of anthrax.

Cutaneous anthrax

- The most common naturally occurring type of infection (> 95% of cases) occurring most often after skin contact with contaminated meat, wool, hides, or leather from infected animals, usually after the bacterium enters via a cut or abrasion.
- Incubation period of 1 to 12 days.
- Infection begins as a raised bump that resembles a spider bite, then within 24 to 48 hours it develops into a vesicle, and finally a painless ulcer, usually 1 to 3 cm in diameter, with a characteristic black necrotic area in the center. Although the lesion is typically painless, the patient may experience fever, malaise, and headache.
- Lymph glands adjacent to the infected area may swell.
- About 20% of untreated patients die. Deaths are rare if patient is given appropriate antimicrobial therapy.

Inhalation anthrax

- The most lethal form of anthrax.
- Anthrax spores must be aerosolized in order to cause inhalational anthrax.
- The incubation period is not clear: It may be 1 to 7 days, possibly up to 2 months.
- Resembling a viral respiratory illness, initial symptoms include sore throat, mild fever, muscle aches, and malaise.
- Symptoms may progress to respiratory failure and shock with meningitis developing frequently.
- A runny nose is a rare symptom of inhalation anthrax. If the patient has a runny nose with other common flu-like symptoms, he probably does not have anthrax
- Most people with inhalation anthrax have high WBC counts and no increase in the number of lymphocytes.
- All patients with inhalation anthrax show an abnormality in their chest X-ray, although, for some patients, the changes may be subtle.
- The case-fatality estimate which is based on incomplete information is about 75%, even with all possible supportive care including appropriate antibiotics.
- The impact on survival of a delay in post-exposure prophylaxis or treatment isn't known.

Gastrointestinal anthrax

- Usually follows the consumption of raw or undercooked contaminated meat.
- Incubation period of 1 to 7 days.
- Associated with severe abdominal distress followed by fever and signs of septicemia.
- The disease can take an oropharyngeal or abdominal form.
- Involvement of the oropharynx is usually characterized by lesions at the base of the tongue, sore throat, difficulty swallowing, fever, and swollen lymph glands.
- Involvement of the bowel usually causes nausea, loss of appetite, vomiting, and fever, followed by abdominal pain, vomiting blood, and bloody diarrhea.
- The case-fatality estimate is 25% to 60%, but the effect of early antibiotic treatment on that estimate isn't known.

Index

t refers to a table.

t refers to a table.

B

t refers to a table.

t refers to a table.

t refers to a table.

t refers to a table.

t refers to a table.

t refers to a table.

t refers to a table.

t refers to a table.

t refers to a table.

t refers to a table.

t refers to a table.

t refers to a table.

t refers to a table.

t refers to a table.

t refers to a table.

T

t refers to a table.

t refers to a table.

t refers to a table.